Elisabeth BRETON

Reflex relaxation and back stimulation techniques

Elisabeth BRETON

Reflex relaxation and back stimulation techniques

The back, an emotional storage area

ScienciaScripts

Imprint
Any brand names and product names mentioned in this book are subject to trademark, brand or patent protection and are trademarks or registered trademarks of their respective holders. The use of brand names, product names, common names, trade names, product descriptions etc. even without a particular marking in this work is in no way to be construed to mean that such names may be regarded as unrestricted in respect of trademark and brand protection legislation and could thus be used by anyone.

Cover image: www.ingimage.com

This book is a translation from the original published under ISBN 978-620-6-72616-6.

Publisher:
Sciencia Scripts
is a trademark of
Dodo Books Indian Ocean Ltd. and OmniScriptum S.R.L publishing group

120 High Road, East Finchley, London, N2 9ED, United Kingdom
Str. Armeneasca 28/1, office 1, Chisinau MD-2012, Republic of Moldova, Europe
Printed at: see last page
ISBN: 978-620-8-23047-0

REFLEX TECHNIQUES

RELAXATION AND BACK STIMULATION

The back, an emotional storage area

I dedicate this book to my two teachers, Albert Debouté, an osteopath in Paris, and Raymond Richard (1942-2011), founder of the *Richard Osteopathic Research Institute* (R.O.R.I) and author of several books, whom I had the pleasure of meeting during my osteopathic studies in 2007, and who gave me so much.

They were passionate about sharing and passing on high-quality teaching that I've been applying ever since, adapting certain reflex techniques to massages aimed at well-being and stress management.

The year I spent at R.O.R.I. will always be engraved in my memory! These lessons enriched my vision of the reflexology profession and greatly evolved my practice of reflexology, which I discovered in 1998.

Thanks to them, I have developed a specific method: "Conjunctive, periosteal and viscerocutaneous dermalgia reflex techniques (osteopathic contribution to reflexology)® - trademark registered with the INPI on 23/01/2019, under N°4517964.

"Study, not to know more, but to know better".
Seneca

CONTENTS

PREFACE

5

I'm delighted and honoured to be taking part in Elisabeth Breton's foreword on the treatment of the back as seen through the eyes of a seasoned reflexologist. As she jokingly told me, all she had left was her back... I invite you to discover her vision, her experience and her ability to synthesise clear, practical protocols. A specific method designed to relax local tensions, as well as those accumulated over the years by stress and emotions.

It's an approach that will complement everyone's experience and offer a different approach to the back. And as an old Latin proverb says, "scratch my back and I'll scratch yours".

Enjoy your reading.

Joakim VALÉRO

Emergency doctor, specialising in stress management

Author of "Ma remise en forme en un week-end" - First Edition
Co-author of "Le stress, ça vous parle? Understanding its history and mechanisms" - Edition Vie
And "Réflexologie et troubles fonctionnels: Prise en charge et gestion du stress par les techniques reflexes" - published by DUNOD

<u>FOREWORD</u>

I wrote my first book on "*Reflexology for fitness and well-being*" in 2014, published by Editions Vie . [1]

Writing this book had been on my mind for quite some time. Buoyed by the encouragement of my practitioners, the desire to share my experiences and my knowledge of stress and associated functional disorders, and following on from my previous publications, I finally took the time to summarise my courses on this subject... the back, that part of the body which absorbs so much emotional stress!

The first time I gave a talk on the '*Back, an area of emotional storage*' was in 2004, at an alternative medicine fair in Paris. It was rated by journalists and the general public as the best lecture in the 'body/mind' category.

And now it's been 20 years!

The information provided in this book is for information purposes only and is the fruit of many years' work.

They are in no way a substitute for the teaching offered at my Professional Training Centre, nor are they intended to be a substitute for a consultation, a medical procedure or a prescription for medication.

They can in no way replace the advice of a doctor or other health professional.

---

[1] Reflexology for fitness and well-being / 978-3-639-68621-0 / 9783639686210 / 3639686217 (editions-vie.com)

<u>ACKNOWLEDGEMENTS</u>

I would like to thank all those who have contributed in one way or another to the production of this book, and in particular the people I have met throughout my professional career as a reflexologist.

I've had the pleasure of accompanying them through different stages of their lives, relieving their tensions and emotions, and helping them to feel better and feel good.

I'd also like to thank all the practitioners I've had the pleasure of training in these techniques. I'm delighted to have been able to share my experiences with them, and to have been able to provide them with new skills for better care of people who are said to be under stress.

With all my gratitude

Elisabeth Breton

"Health is a state of complete physical, mental and social well-being and not merely the absence of disease or infirmity.[2]

---

[2] Definition of health by the World Health Organisation in 1948.

INTRODUCTION

The human body is made up of different systems or apparatus: respiratory, digestive, cardiovascular, nervous, lymphatic, muscular, bone.... Under stress, these systems and their functions can be disrupted, leading to pain and disorders.

Directly or indirectly, the use of reflex techniques affects each of these metabolic functions, as reflex massage considerably reduces the harmful effects of stress.

A state of stress arises when our body feels attacked by a situation that is difficult to manage, whether internal or external.

Stress is a set of neuro-psychological reactions designed to maintain balance in the face of an external agent.

Stress can manifest itself both physically and psychologically, and systematically generates a hyperfunction of the nervous system, which in turn is linked to all the organs and tissues of the body. As the nervous system is closely linked to the hormonal system, a cascade of chemical reactions is triggered, leading to obvious disorders. The functional disorder reflects a dysfunction in the body.

The term "functional disorder" covers all symptoms that have no clearly identified medical cause.

Psychological factors, including emotional stress, can predispose, precipitate or aggravate back pain. They encourage the onset of chronicity and form part of the psychosocial indicators known as "yellow flags".

Stress causes hyperfunction of the nervous system and hypertonicity of the musculoskeletal system, particularly in the back. **This area, which is linked to the dermatomes, is hypersensitive to reflex stimulation**.

When a muscle is tense or stiffened by stress or injury, it contracts. This contraction compresses and reduces blood flow to the muscle. The dried muscle fibres stick together. In more serious cases, waste products and toxins accumulate in the muscle fibres and develop points of tension or "*knots*", which resemble hard pebbles lodged deep in the muscle. Calcium deposits can form.

Nerve tension and muscle contraction have an effect on the bone system, causing increased pain and reduced mobility. Many tensions can be caused by poor posture, mechanical problems (articular, musculoskeletal), poor vascularisation (congested tissue) or stress.

Reflex massage relaxes a contracted muscle, increasing blood flow and encouraging muscle fibres to separate. Toxins and waste products are then expelled from the cells and eliminated in the urine, faeces or sweat. Improved blood circulation relieves many muscular pains and tensions.

The reflex techniques applied in reflex massage act on the different levels of tension, inducing a state of muscular, tissue and emotional relaxation and activating better microcirculation.

Stimulation of the **muscular and ligament receptors** in the different muscle layers of the back, as well as the various **skin corpuscles**, leads to muscle relaxation and the secretion of feel-good hormones (endorphin, dopamine, etc.).

Reflex techniques for the connective tissue of the back aim to :

> ➢ reduce sympathetic hyperactivity in functional disorders, joint and muscle pain, etc.
> ➢ drain connective tissue and decongest the area locally (derivative effect)
> ➢ restore and maintain metabolic balance.

I think it's very important to stress that the relaxation reflex massage and back tension due to stress that I cover in this book should not be confused with the manual treatment of a physiotherapist for a painful myofascial syndrome (MDS). Although a practitioner may touch an area affected by MDS, he or she will not treat it in the same way as a physiotherapist.

Several authors describe MDS as a functional, reversible and above all painful disturbance of the musculoskeletal system.

It is characterised by several symptoms, the main one being myofascial pain. This pain is due to myofascial trigger points, also known as Trigger Points. These are small, hypersensitive areas in the skeletal muscle, located in one or more taut bands, causing pain on palpation and reproducing the pain symptoms known and felt by the patient[3] . The onset is often insidious, due to acute or chronic mechanical and/or muscular stress .[4]

---

[3] Borg-Stein J, Simons DG. Myofascial pain. Arch Phys Med Rehabil. March 2002;83:S40-7.
[4] "Le traitement manuel du Syndrome Myofascial Douloureux à travers la littérature", dissertation by Mathilde VAUTRIN memoires.kine-nancy.eu/vautrin2017.pdf

Numerous studies and books on "reflex massage" have been published since the beginning of the 20th century [e5] .

Reflex massages have long been practised by chiropractors, osteopaths and physiotherapists.

In 1930, Franck Chapman, an American chiropractor, observed that sluggish lymphatic flow led to physical dysfunction. He established a series of lymphatic reflex points, the stimulation of which improved his patients' health.

George Goodheart, a chiropractor best known for his work on applied kinesiology in the 1960s, took his research further and associated Chapman points with muscles. He observed that stimulation of the Chapman points could strengthen or relax a muscle.

In his book "*Health through Touch*", American chiropractor John Thie calls Chapman's points *"Neurolymphatic reflex points*" and draws up a map of these points on the body.

Several German doctors have contributed to the development of work on connective tissue, including :
Wolfgang Kohlrausch, author of several works on reflex zones: "*Les rapports réciproques réflexes entre les organes internes et les muscles squelettiques et leur usage thérapeutique*" (1937). "*Reflex zones in the skin, subcutaneous tissue and muscles*" (1953). "*Basics of reflex zone

---

⁵ "Reflexology for fitness and well-being", E.Breton, Editions Vie (2014)

massage" (1956). "*Reflex zone massage in the musculature and connective tissue*" (1961).

Teirich-Leube, author of "*Massage of reflex zones in connective tissue in rheumatic diseases and diseases of the* internal *organs*" (1952).

Elisabeth Dicke, a German physiotherapist, published "*My connective tissue massage*" in 1958.

In France, osteopath Raymond Richard (1942-2011), author of 12 books translated into several languages, including the manual on "*Techniques réflexes conjonctives, périostées et dermalgies viscéro-cutanées*" published in 2001, presents a synthetic study of connective tissue, based on research by German and Austrian authors.

I had the honour of meeting him and learning a few reflex techniques that I was then able to adapt to reflexology massage with his permission.[6]

Relaxation reflex massage can in no way be equated with medical care, physiotherapy or osteopathy.
It promotes well-being through physical relaxation and stress-relief.

---

[6] Réflexologie et troubles fonctionnels - Prise en charge et gestion du stress par les techniques réflexes - Book and ebook Complementary Therapies by Elisabeth Breton - Dunod

"Every gesture is a word from the body whose phrases are postures. "
Joseph **_Messinger_**

PART ONE: ANATOMY OF THE BACK

In order to better approach reflex massage of the back, it is essential and necessary to acquire a basic knowledge of anatomy and physiology, to better understand how our body functions, our systems, their interactions and any disturbances.

Anatomy (from the Greek word *anatomé* meaning "to dissect") is the study of the structure of the different parts of the body and their interrelationships.

Physiology (from the Greek words *phusis*, "nature" and *logos*, "science") studies the "dynamic" functioning of the human body, from the level of chemical organisation to that of the organism.

Pathology studies the malfunctions of anatomical structures and physiological mechanisms, which are at the root of the countless diseases that can affect the proper functioning of the human body.

Functional disorders are symptoms that have no clearly identified medical cause.

The maintenance of life depends on the correct synergistic functioning of eleven systems: cardiovascular, endocrine, nervous, respiratory, digestive, integumentary, muscular, bone, urinary, lymphatic and genital. These systems work in close collaboration to ensure the major functions of life.

There is a relative "internal stability", responding to the incessant variations in the external environment. The term "homeostasis" defines this stability of the internal environment.

Initially defined by Claude Bernard[7] in the 19th century, then developed by Walter Bradfort Cannon[8] at the beginning of the 20th century, the term *homeostasis* comes from the Greek *hómoios*, "similar", and *stásis*, "place where something stands".

As far as reflex massage is concerned, I'd use the term 'balance' to describe adaptation and reflex self-regulation.

Considering human health to be intimately linked to its environment, the field of stress prevention and management takes great care to detect external stress factors, which are major causes of many illnesses. Health is a state of balance between the physical body and the mind, and between the human being and his or her natural and social environment. To be in good health is not just to be free of disease, but also to be able to acquire the resources that provide a sense of well-being and vitality, and to enjoy an optimal quality of life. It means learning to respect optimal living conditions to avoid disease (hygiene, prevention) by limiting environmental stress factors.

Recommendations on how to take stress into account when supporting people come from learned societies such as the World Health Organisation[9] or the French National Authority for Health (HAS) . [10]

---

[7] Claude Bernard, *Introduction to the study of experimental medicine*, 1865
[8] Walter Cannon, *The Wisdom of the Body*, 1932, p. 177-201
[9] WHO recommendation: www.who.int/fr/publications-detail.
[10] HAS recommendation: www.has-sante.fr

Relaxation and reflexology fall within the scope of prevention, sustainable health and personal well-being.

17

The musculoskeletal system of the back

Three distinct systems - **the skeleton, the muscles and the nerves** - are necessary for the back to play its role properly. All it takes is for one of these systems to be affected to cause pain and disabling stiffness. Back pain is very often caused by the way we sit, stand or walk. Posture is a very individual problem.

Considered "the disease of the century", back pain affects many people in France and around the world. According to Assurance Maladie figures, musculoskeletal disorders account for almost 90% of occupational illnesses in France, and back pain accounts for 20% of accidents at work.

The results of a survey carried out in France in November 2023 by Statista's Consumer Insights[11] show that back pain is, along with headache, the most common physical pain among French adults.

Pain is the body's alarm system. Sometimes, however, the pain seems to originate in a different part of the body from the source of the pain. A large percentage of musculoskeletal disorders (MSDs) are due to poor 'adaptation' to nervous tension and stress.

Hardened areas or points" are small regions of muscle that remain chronically contracted, which can appear after an injury, poor posture habits or even following a state of anxiety or strong emotion. The muscle fibres are then in a state of permanent spasm and often radiate pain to distant areas.

---

[11] Graph: Back pain: the "disease of the century" | Statista

In some cases, the physical and emotional stress is so intense that **"myogelosis"** can occur.

This term appeared in Max Lange's accounts in 1931. He used the term "myogelosis" to describe "muscle hardening", the idea being that muscle protein "gels"[12] . The hypothesis was that muscle contraction was due to colloidal gelation of the muscle substance. For a long time, the term "myogelosis" was associated with trigger points in German literature.

I first heard about 'myogeloses' in Serbia, at the Banja Koviljaca spa[13] , with which I had a partnership. Reflexology is a recognised discipline and is integrated into their health system.
From 2006 to 2011, I organised a number of trips for my association "La Fontaine du Bien-être"[14] , for my clients and practitioners. We discussed different practices with the medical team and health professionals at their medical SPA, where we also benefit from wellness cures. They take a very holistic approach.
The word holistic comes from the Greek holos meaning whole, entire. Thus, the holistic approach consists of taking into account a person as a whole, rather than looking at him or her in a compartmentalised way.

I learnt a lot from them and this made me want to train in osteopathy. I did so in 2007, when I enrolled on the Reflex Techniques course at the R.O.R.I. (Richard Osteopathic Research Institute).

Many people experience discomfort or pain in their back which may be triggered by a chronic muscle contracture in the jaw, neck or shoulders,

---

[12] Lange M. Die Muskelhärten (Myogelosen). Munich: J.F. Lehmann's Verlag; 1931
[13] Specijalna bolnica Banja Koviljača (banjakoviljaca.rs)
[14] La Fontaine du Bien-Être - Association of reflexology practitioners (fontainedubienetre.fr)

as a result of stress-related tension, of which they are completely unaware. In this type of reaction, the trigger point remains 'silent' until it is revealed by the reflex massage touch.

Back pain has a wide variety of causes (physical, organic, genetic, emotional).

These days, health problems are very often linked to **stress.** A well-rested person suffers less from exhaustion and fatigue, and is less sensitive to stress. Stress is also a major factor in the onset or amplification of pain.

Knowing how to "manage" stress, in particular through relaxation exercises based on breathing and muscle relaxation, can in some cases break the vicious circle of "*stress-muscle tension-pain*".

Projected back pain can also be caused by :
- Lung problems
- Heart problems
- Kidney problems (kidney stones)
- Bladder problems
- Gynaecological problems
- Inflammation of the pancreas
- An ulcer of the duodenum or stomach

Back pain can be caused by a variety of events. The vertebrae may fracture following a violent blow (accident, fall). Muscles can contract or even tear as a result of over-exertion. Other injuries can result from years of manual labour. The back can also be affected by a degenerative disease, a neurological problem, a bone deformity or simply be weakened during growth. Back pain can also be symptomatic of many other problems.

Stress is a daily source that affects the neuro-musculo-skeletal system. Daily worries, poor posture and repeated trauma are all factors that weaken the back, creating tension and various types of pain (neck, region between the shoulder blades, lumbar region). Initially temporary, the pain can become chronic.

CAUTION: The practitioner must be sure that back tension is caused by stress as a functional disorder. If in doubt, the practitioner should refrain from treating the problem and encourage the patient to consult a health professional (doctor, physiotherapist, osteopath, etc.).

I've sometimes refused to apply a reflex massage to the back if I noticed that the person was showing signs of excessive stiffness (in the neck, for example, or elsewhere), especially if they hadn't consulted a doctor beforehand and hadn't undergone any tests (x-rays, etc.). In a similar case, I suggested foot reflexology to the patient, while waiting for the results to rule out any doubt or possible contraindication to reflex massage of the back. In this particular case, the person followed my advice and informed me a few days after our conversation that she had had a consultation and an X-ray, which revealed a herniated cervical disc, which could explain the stiffness in her neck and the lack of mobility in her cervical vertebrae.

You should always be very careful when it comes to reflex massages of the body, especially those of the back, even if their aim is simply to relax the body.

<h1 style="text-align:center"><u>The spine or rachis</u></h1>

The human skeleton comprises more than **206 bones**, more than half of which are located in the hands and feet.

Bone is a living, spongy tissue, a "hard" connective tissue. Osteoblasts are the bone-producing cells.

Osteoclasts destroy (or resorb) bone, enabling it to maintain its shape and mechanical qualities.

Osteoblasts and osteoclasts ensure ongoing bone remodelling.

The spinal column, a fundamental part of the architectural organisation of the human body, is a living whole that responds and adapts to the different needs of life.

The spine is subject to the constraints of gravity. The human centre of gravity is located around the umbilicus. Gravity forces the back muscles to contract constantly. In this way, the vertebrae are constantly adapting in order to escape the constraints of gravity.

The spinal column, also known as the rachis, is made up of thirty-three bony parts or vertebrae. These vertebrae have certain characteristics in common, and others that vary according to their location.

These parts are held together by the elastic structure and physiological tone of the small muscles and ligaments that hold them together.

The whole system, which is highly flexible, is controlled by nerve centres in the spinal cord, which travels up to the brain along the vertebral canal in the centre of the spinal column, where it is protected.

<u>Composition of the spinal column :</u>

A. **Cervical: 7 vertebrae** which allow movement of the head and neck.
B. **Dorsal curvature: 12 vertebrae** which allow the torsional movements of the trunk. The ribs are attached to the costal facets.

C. **Lumbar curvature: 5 vertebrae** which allow flexion and torsion movements.

D. **Sacral curvature: 5 fused vertebrae**; supporting the spinal column, they are attached to the pelvis.

E. **Coccyx: 4 fused vertebrae**, the remains of a tail.

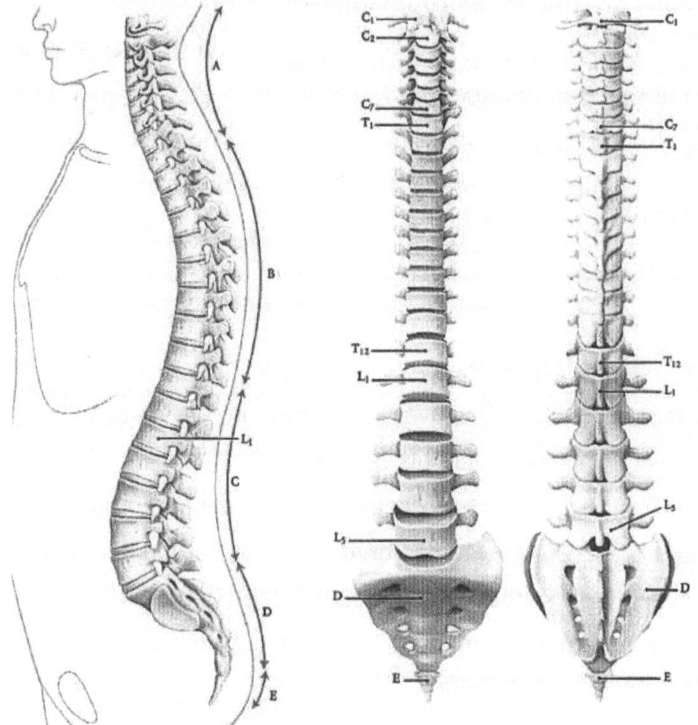

Drawing Institut R.O.R.I.

The vertebrae overlap to form the spinal canal, into which the spinal cord descends.

Each vertebra has two main parts: **the** solid **vertebral body** at the front and the **posterior arch at** the back, which protects the spinal cord.

The vertebrae are linked together and separated by **intervertebral discs.** They are held in place by ligaments and muscles. There is a **fibrous disc** between each vertebra, which gives the spine its flexibility and mobility. The intervertebral disc is made up of shock-absorbing cartilage.

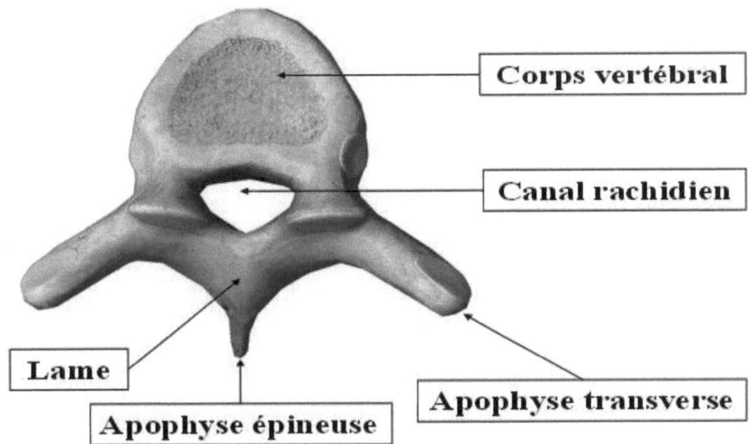

Source Visible Body

The human spine has 23 intervertebral discs.

This shock-absorbing disc has a gelatinous nucleus at its centre, called the *nucleus pulposus*, and is surrounded by a fibrous ring that prevents the disc from sliding towards the spinal canal and restricting the passage of the spinal nerve.

The disc that separates the 5th or last lumbar vertebra from the 1st sacrum vertebra is the most fragile. This weakness is aggravated by professional and sporting activities, reckless effort, age and the absence of tonic muscles. This disc thins more at the back than at the front under the effect of the mechanical load it bears.

To a lesser degree, but for the same reasons, the discs between the 5 and 4 or between the 4 and 3 V. Lumbar also become thinner. To avoid damaging your vertebrae, you need to stand up straight, develop your back and abdominal muscles, and avoid lifting objects that are too heavy.

<u>Important role of certain vertebrae</u>:

> **T12 or D12** = <u>the dorsolumbar hinge vertebra</u> It is a transition vertebra. This dorsolumbar hinge accumulates numerous compensations. It is built for flexion-extension, is very sensitive to rotation and has no protection against lateral translation.

> **L3** = this is the only vertebra with parallel vertebral plates; it is <u>the base that supports the entire spine</u>.
> It acts as a muscular relay between the iliacus and the thoracic spine. This explains the frequency of injuries to this vertebra.

Each vertebra is the starting point of a muscular tendon, a branch of the central nervous system linked to the skin, muscles and organs of an area of the body called a ***metamerus*,** and corresponds to ganglia of the sympathetic nervous system which controls contractions and relaxations.

Any deformation of a vertebra will have an influence by creating tension or a blockage (reduction in circulation) in the neighbouring area, and therefore the nerves and muscles.

The constant pressure exerted on the spine and back muscles makes this part of the body more fragile.

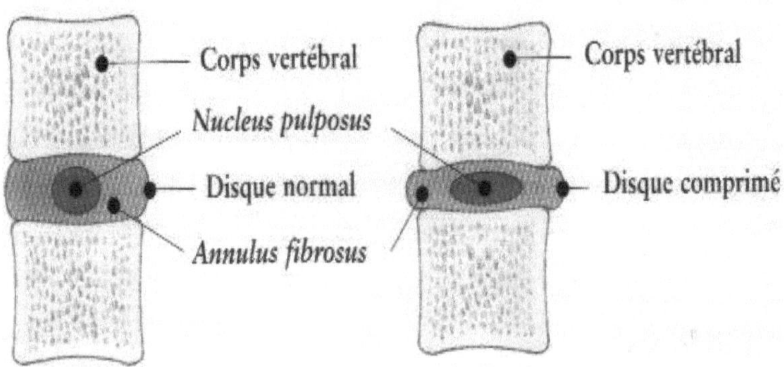

Drawing osteopathy course Institut R.O.R.I.

The spinal column has 149 joints: some connect the vertebrae to each other, others connect the spinal column to other parts of the skeleton (base of the skull, ribs, sacroiliac joints, hip joints).

The body's joints are held together and strengthened by ligaments.
- Longitudinal ligaments
- Intervertebral ligaments
- The iliolumbar ligaments (they attach the lumbar vertebrae L4/L5 to the iliac crest and the sacrum, and play a major role in protecting the last two lumbar discs).
- The sacroiliac ligaments (they are not part of the ligaments of the lumbar region, but their pathology classifies them among the causes of low back pain)

If they were not supported by the structure formed by the joints, ligaments and discs, the vertebrae of the spine would rub painfully against each other.

The joints, with their ligamentary and muscular dependencies, are rich in **sensory sensors**.

The muscles and bones of the body form the musculoskeletal system, which shapes, supports and enables us to perform mechanical tasks such as walking, talking, standing up straight or sitting down.

This system is sensitive to overactivity, susceptible to injury and inflammation, and is a frequent source of pain.

Musculoskeletal pain is rarely caused by bones, unless they are broken or in poor condition. The cause of the pain is to be found in the muscles and the tissues that connect them (tendons and ligaments), and more specifically in the joints. Hard-working joints such as those in the neck, back, hips, arms and legs, as well as the knee - the most complex joint in the body - are likely to be largely responsible for the problem.

The two belts

The limb girdles are the bony and articular assemblies that attach the limbs to the trunk.

At the top, located at the top of the ribs, **the shoulder girdle** is formed by the sternum at the front and in the middle, the two clavicles at the front and the two shoulder blades at the back.
It connects the upper limbs to the trunk. It is characterised by its *mobility*.
It is not articularly linked to the spinal column, but to the thoracic cage.

At the bottom of the trunk**, the pelvic girdle**, or **pelvis**, is formed by the sacrum and the two iliac bones.
It connects the lower limbs to the trunk. The joints between these bones are not very mobile, which gives it a characteristic *stability*. This belt is connected to the trunk by the sacro-lumbar joint, which joins it to the spinal column. But it is also the place where the femurs articulate with the trunk: *the pelvis is thus a pressure-transmitting element.*
These pressures are due to the weight of the body and counter-pressures coming from the ground via the lower limbs.

The muscles and fascias of the back

A powerful musculature holds, contains and joins the vertebrae together, one above the other, to form the longitudinal vertebral axis, which is both rigid and flexible, capable of supporting the trunk and ensuring upright posture and balance.

The back muscles are arranged in layers (or planes):

- ➢ Surface plane
- ➢ Medium (or intermediate) plan
- ➢ Deep plane

Superior plane: superficial muscles, such as the scapula lift, trapezius, latissimus dorsi and rhomboids.

Beneath this layer lie long, thong-like muscles such as the long dorsal muscle of the thorax, which is used for bending, straightening and rotating the trunk.

Middle plane: posterior superior and posterior inferior small serratus muscles. Their motor action is related to respiration: elevation of the ribs (inspiration) and lowering of the ribs (expiration).

Deep plane (these are the muscles of the vertebral gutter): longissimus muscles of the head, neck and thorax, spinal muscles (spinous, ilio-costal, multifidus muscles), quadratus lumborum muscle.

These muscles help stabilise the spine (extension and inclination of the cervical, thoracic and lumbar spine, and extension of the trunk).

The deepest layer is made up of thick, short muscles which connect each vertebra in pairs or sometimes cover several vertebrae. Above this layer, long, strap-like muscles, mostly attached to the back of the pelvis, fan out towards the head to attach to the ribs and vertebrae.

Reflex relaxation of the back gradually relaxes these muscle layers, from the superficial to the deep layers. Tissue relaxation is progressive.

<u>The back muscles are supported by the abdominal muscles.</u>

The stomach contains abdominal muscles, which are divided into several groups with specific functions:

> **The rectus abdominis**: the rectus abdominis is a muscle that runs from the sternum to the pubis. It looks like a chocolate bar because it is made up of several squares which, when you are muscular, can be felt under the skin. This muscle flexes the trunk.

> **The transverse** muscle: the transverse muscle is found in the depths of the abdomen. It acts during the contraction and allows the stomach to be drawn in.

> **The large oblique and the small oblique**: these muscles are located on the side of the stomach. The lesser oblique lies under the greater oblique. They contract and allow the body to twist.

Plan superficiel

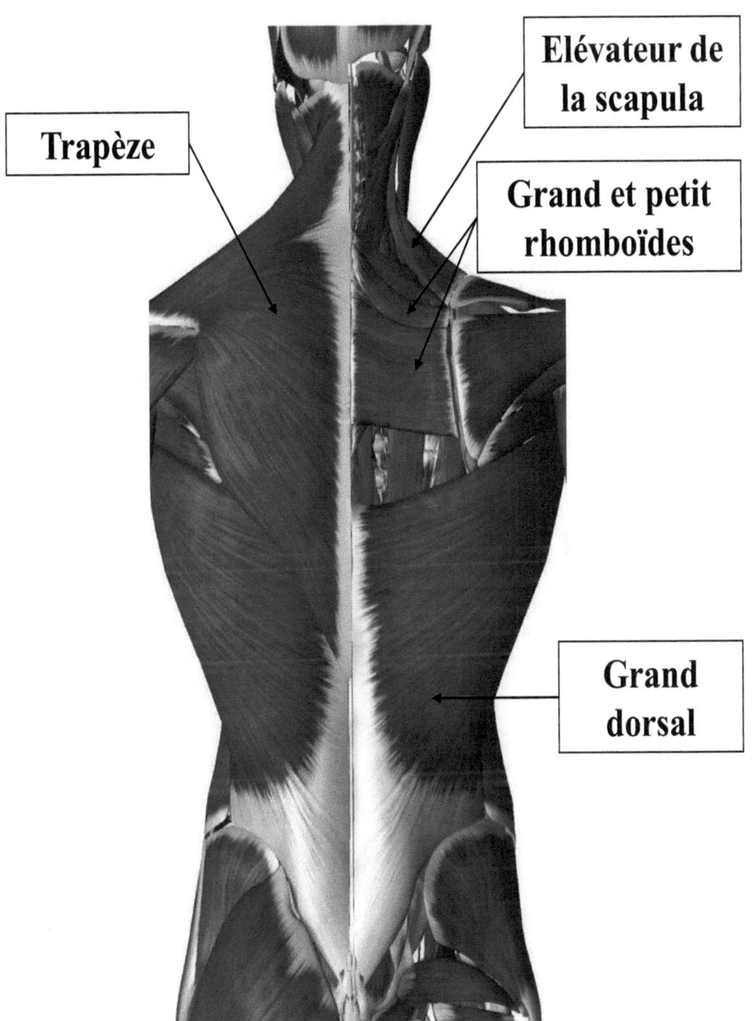

<u>Muscles superficiels</u> : élévateur de la scapula, le trapèze, le grand dorsal et les rhomboïdes.

Plan moyen ou intermédiaire

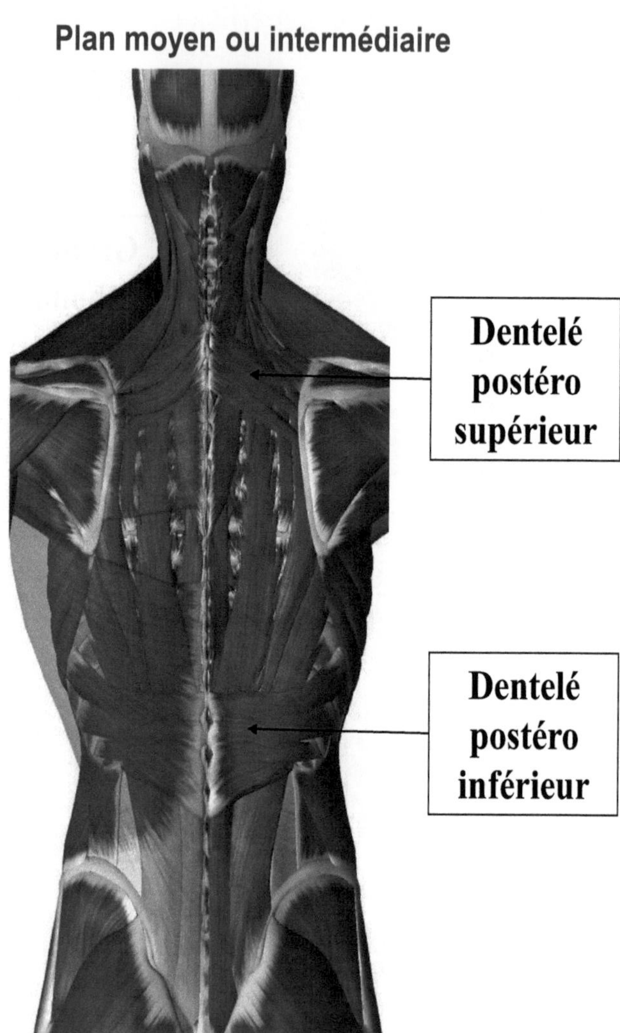

<u>Muscles moyens</u> : muscles petit dentelé postéro supérieur et postéro inférieur.

Deep muscles: longissimus muscles of the head, neck and thorax, spinal muscles (spinatus, ilio-costalis, multifidus muscles), quadratus lumborum muscle.

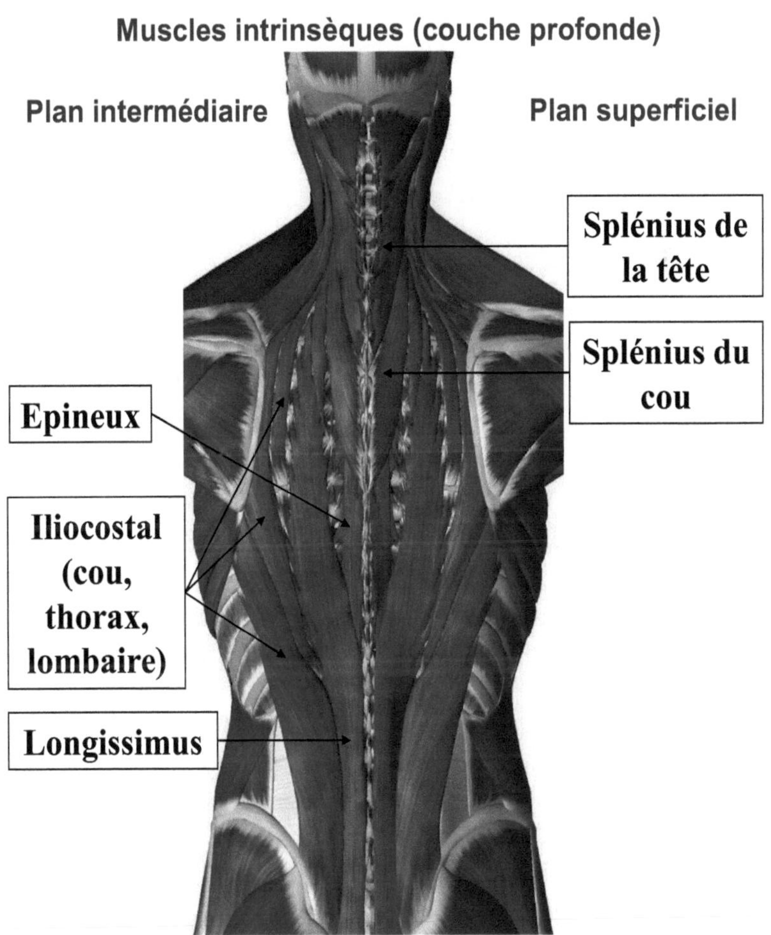

Muscles intermédiaires de la couche profonde : muscles longissimus, iliocostal (des lombes, du thorax et du cou) et épineux.

Muscles superficiels de la couche profonde : splénius de la tête et du cou.

Muscles intrinsèques (couche profonde)

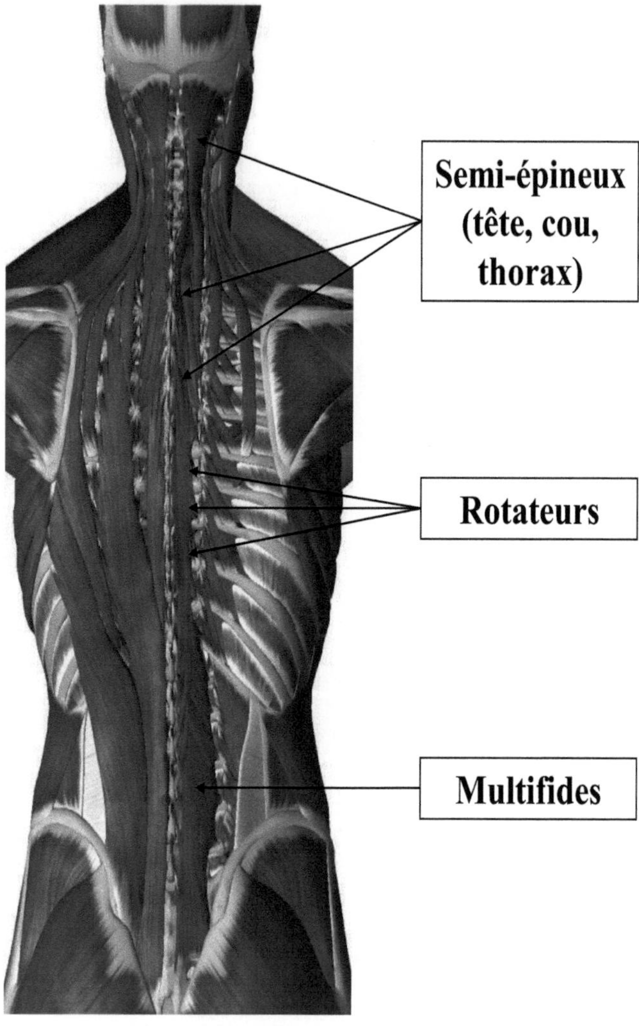

Muscles profonds : Les muscles semi-épineux de la tête, du cou et du thorax, les multifides et les rotateurs.

<u>Muscle tone</u>

Even at rest, a muscle remains slightly contracted: this is the phenomenon of muscle tone, independent of willpower. This phenomenon involves proprioceptors in the muscles and tendons. This permanent "mini-contraction" is due to the activation of certain motor units, which are then taken over by others while the first "rest". Muscle tone does not produce any movement, but keeps the muscle "awake", ready to respond to any stimulation.[15]

<u>Muscular fatigue</u>

Muscular fatigue, following prolonged or excessive effort, defines the muscle's inability to contract, despite continued stimulation. It is linked to the depletion of adenosine triphosphate (ATP) reserves. ATP provides the energy required for chemical reactions in metabolism, locomotion and cell division.

<u>Muscle recovery</u>

After muscular effort, especially if it has been to the point of fatigue, the muscle must recover, i.e. replenish its stocks of glycogen, oxygen (O2) and adenosine triphosphate (ATP), and metabolise excess lactic acid. Muscle recovery corresponds to the repayment of the oxygen debt and the replenishment of ATP stocks.

Reflex massage of the back has multiple beneficial effects on recovery and the restoration of tissue and muscle reflexes.

<u>The fascias of the back</u>

---

[15] *"Le corps humain pour les nuls"* Dr P. Gepner, First Edition, 2009.

A fascia is a fibrous membrane that covers or envelops an anatomical structure. It is a dense connective tissue, very rich in collagen fibres, which forms a sort of sheath.

<u>This fibrous membrane forms a complex network which</u> :

-       Wraps and separates muscles

-       Provides sheaths for nerves and tendons

-       Forms or strengthens ligaments around joints

-       Envelope for various organs and glands

-       Bind all the structures together.

Here are some of the fascias of the back:

1.   <u>Infraspinatus fascia </u>(the infraspinatus muscle is a muscle in the shoulder girdle and forms part of the rotator cuff. In many people, it is tight, and can cause local pain that "burns" at the level of the shoulder blade. The pain can radiate to the neck, shoulders and upper arm).

2.   <u>Thoracolumbar fascia </u>(lumbar fascia covering the deep muscles of the back and trunk. This fascia is essential for the organisation and function of the various muscles in this region).

3.   <u>Lumbosacral fascia </u>(the lumbosacral fascia is a large diamond-shaped sheet which forms part of the deep fascia. Highly developed in the lumbar region, it is made up of several layers of crossed collagen fibres that cover the back muscles in the lower thoracic and lumbar regions before seeping through these muscles to attach to the sacrum).

4.   <u>Gluteal fascia </u>(Fascia covering the middle muscles of the buttock, located more precisely on the iliac crest, sacrum and coccyx, and extending downwards and forwards through the femoral fascia).

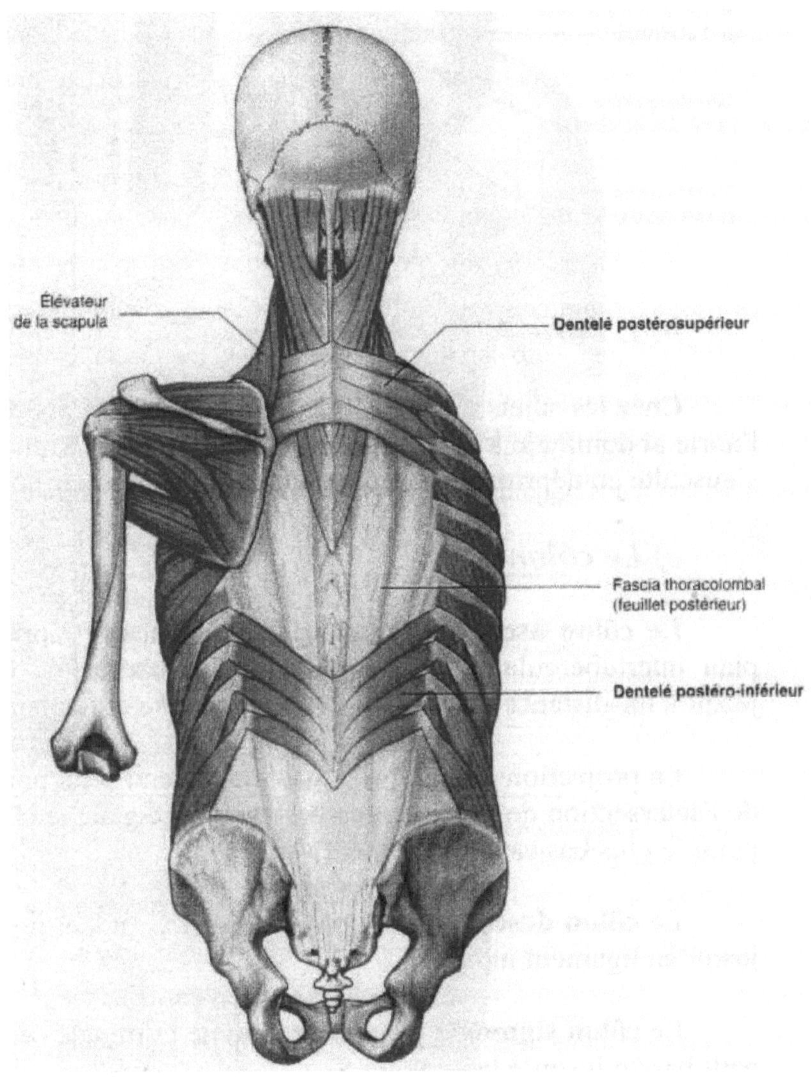

Drawing by the R.O.R.I Institute

The fascia that is omnipresent in the body not only covers all the anatomical parts of the organism, it is also the place of rhythmic animation that ensures the balance between the body and the psyche.

Detecting **connective tissue retraction** requires regular practice, and the practitioner must demonstrate tactile sensitivity, visual acuity and dosage.

Connective tissue is the organ of form, which also makes the body a plastic form. Physiologically, we can consider that there is only one connective tissue in the body, which divides infinitely to ensure the link between all the tissues and their nutrition. In this way, the fascia forms a veritable spider's web that allows tension to be distributed and harmonised at all times, whatever the position of the body.

In Latin, fascia means band or strip. The classic definition, taken from the Flammarion medical dictionary, is as follows: *The fascial envelope of a muscle or region.*

Fascias are particularly sensitive to any disruptive element, such as a physical or psychological shock, an accumulation of stress or intense physical activity. Their supple, elastic and fluid consistency becomes hard, rigid and tense.

Over time, fascias, by tightening, can create knots, blockages and restrictions that disrupt the rhythm and function of the structures they cover, or even compress the nerves or arteries that run through them.

When fascias are stretched, the arteries running through them are partially "strangled", blood flow is slowed and less energy is conveyed. In this case, the tissues or organs concerned suffer and their functions or vitality are disrupted.

Fluid stagnation in the fascia must be avoided. Blood supply depends on the nervous system. Stress can lead to general vasoconstriction; this reaction, which makes the person pale, is accompanied by an intense cold that extends to the very edges of the bone.

Whatever movements we make, our fascias enable us to maintain the fluidity of the movement thanks to their plasticity, and therefore to adapt the proposed deformation without breaking.

The fascia's reaction to stress: tensing, tension, loss of sliding surface, adhesions, cold (vasoconstriction in the bones), desensitisation. Fascia is a memory material. Its behaviour when faced with a new stress depends on its history, i.e. the series of stresses it has received in the past.

Over time, restricted mobility leads to poor vascularisation, dehydration of the bone and sutures, and a form of calcification or densification. Poor irrigation of the nervous system leads to neurological, vascular, hormonal and psychological dysfunction, etc.

Bone, considered hard to the touch, is a tissue that reacts in the same way as muscle or fascia. It loses its flexibility and adaptability when it is subjected to too much stress (which may be physical or emotional). When you use your hands, you feel that the bone is rigid, dry and dense. During reflex massage, the bone gradually regains its malleability (instead of being like a dry sponge, it becomes like a plump, supple, adaptable sponge).

<h1 style="text-align:center"><u>PART TWO: PHYSIOLOGY OF THE BACK</u></h1>

<h2 style="text-align:center"><u>Nerves</u></h2>

Back pain has a wide variety of causes: nerves and the spinal cord can be damaged, leading to severe pain in the arms and legs (sciatica, cervicobrachial neuralgia or arm pain, fibrosis of nerve roots, spinal cord injury).

The nervous system resembles a vast communication network throughout the body. It is made up of fibres and billions of nerve cells or neurons, which detect and process all the information coming from outside or inside the body.

Every second, whether we are awake or asleep, the nerves carry information in the form of **electrical impulses** from different parts of the body to the brain. It is through this complex network of nerves that the brain monitors and controls all bodily functions.

Nerve impulses are transmitted to the muscle cell at the neuromuscular junction, which is **a synapse**.

Starting at the base of the brain and running down the spinal column through the spinal canal, the **spinal cord** is the main relay for information from the nervous system. Over its entire length, it gives rise to nerves which, escaping through the intervertebral spaces, then branch out to form a vast network.

The spinal cord is protected by the meninges and surrounded by the vertebral canal, an empty space within the vertebrae. The spinal nerves, which make up the majority of the peripheral nervous system, originate in the spinal cord. The dorsal roots originate on the posterior side, while the ventral roots originate on the anterior side. When they leave the vertebrae, the spinal nerves divide into branches, which then branch out to innervate the body.

The spinal cord does not run the full length of the spinal column, but breaks off at the first lumbar vertebra (at the base of the back) and continues down the body in **a bundle of nerves known as** the *cauda equina*.

Nerves are divided into two categories:
- > the motor nerves, which transmit messages from the brain to the muscles and glands,
- > the sensory nerves, which send information from the sense organs and the skin to the brain.

There are 31 pairs of spinal nerves:
- > 8 cervical (C1 to C8): innervate the neck and upper limbs.
- > 12 thoracic nerves (T1 to T12): innervate the chest and the upper part of the trunk. The intercostal nerves are located between the ribs.
- > 5 lumbar (L1 to L5): innervate the waist.
- > 5 sacral (S1 to S5): innervate the lower part of the body.
- > 1 coccygeal (Co)
- > Sciatic nerve

Many spinal nerves are grouped **into plexuses,** networks of spinal nerves innervating a specific region.
- > **The cervical plexus** innervates the neck and thoracic cavity.
- > **The brachial plexus** innervates the shoulder girdle and upper limbs.

> **The lumbar and sacral plexuses** innervate the pelvis and lower limbs.

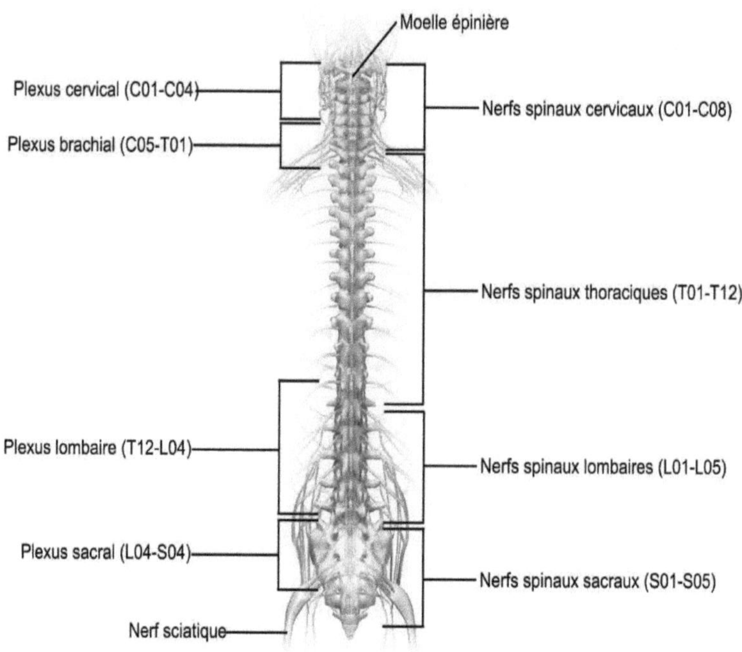

Source Visible Body

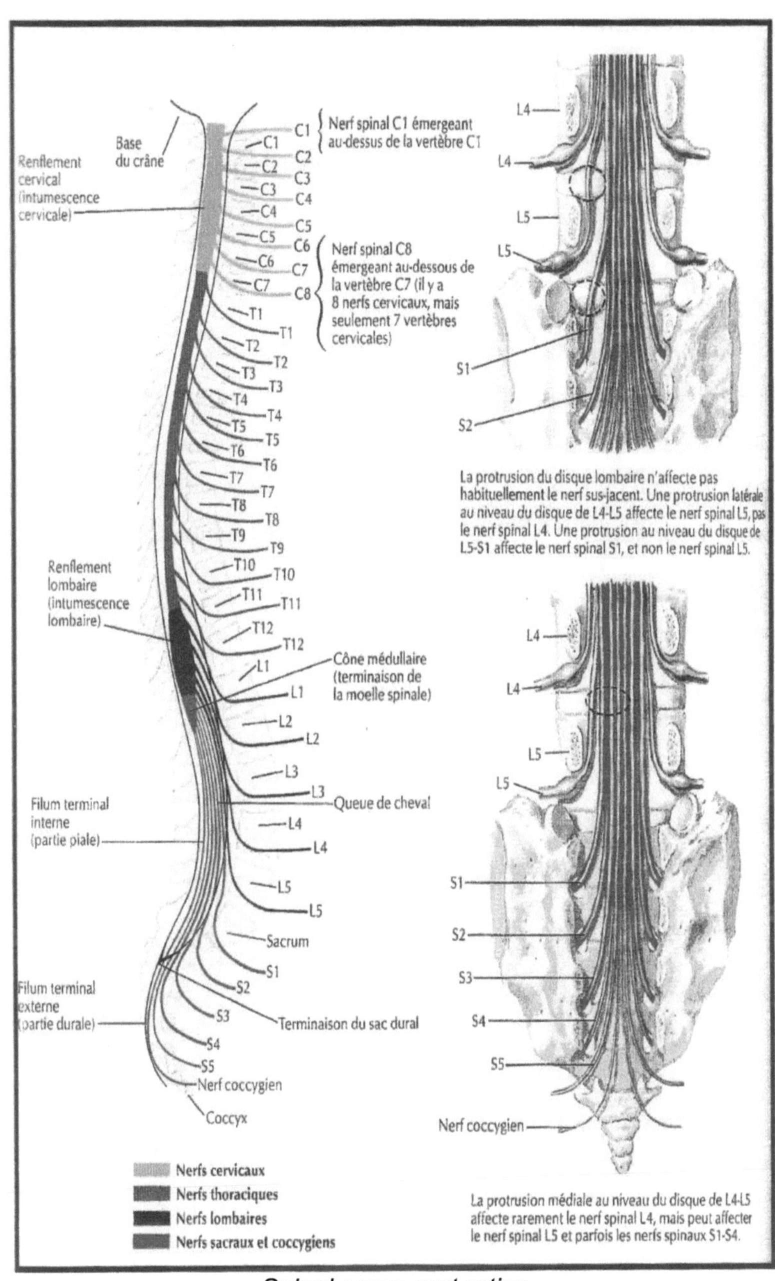

Spinal nerve root ratios
(Drawing by Institut R.O.R.I)

The neurovegetative system is divided into two components:

> <u>Orthosympathetic nervous system</u>, which adapts vital functions to action.

> <u>Parasympathetic nervous system</u>, which ensures recovery, repair and regeneration.

<u>The sympathetic vegetative nervous system</u>

It stimulates the body's functions during periods of intense activity. Sympathetic nerves originate in the thoracic and lumbar segments of the spinal cord. Pre-ganglionic nerve fibres transmit signals from the spinal cord to the ganglia of the sympathetic trunk. After the synapse, they become post-ganglionic fibres and carry the signals to their target organs.

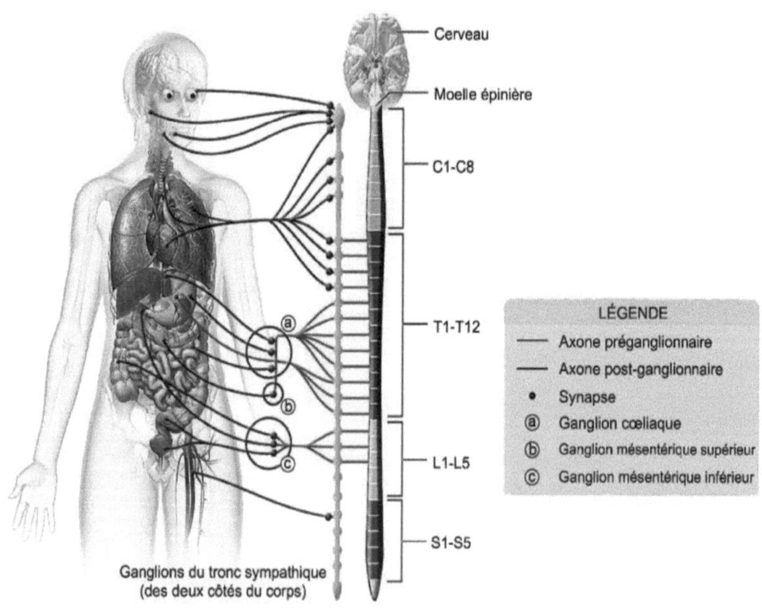

Source Visible Body

<u>**The parasympathetic vegetative nervous system**</u>

It activates resting processes, such as digestion and waste elimination. Parasympathetic nerves originate in the brain stem and sacral spinal cord. Pre-ganglionic nerve fibres synapse with post-ganglionic fibres, which transmit signals to their target organs.

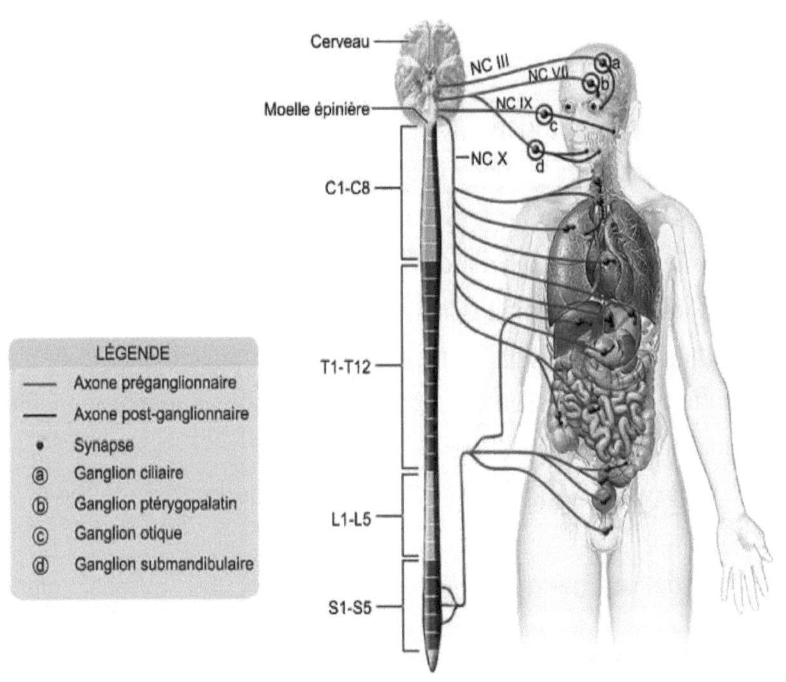

Source : Visible Body

Reflex massages trigger a series of **vegetative reflexes** due to the action on the sympathetic system: nausea, cold sweats, shivering, trembling, etc. These benign side-effects are short-lived.

<u>**The autonomic or vegetative nervous system is composed of several levels:**</u>

a) nerve centres

b) peripheral lymph nodes (paravertebral lymph nodes, pre-visceral lymph nodes and visceral lymph nodes)

c) and fibres.

a)   **Nerve centres** located within the CNS (central nervous system: brain, cerebellum, brain stem, spinal cord).

b) Peripheral lymph nodes

When nerves come together to form bundles at the exit of the spinal cord, this is called a ganglion. A number of these ganglia are located along the outside of the spinal cord and are linked together in the nerve pathway known as the nerve trunk.

The sympathetic nerve trunk runs along the spinal column and has five main ganglia: cervical, celiac (old solar), splanchnic, superior mesenteric and inferior mesenteric.

> **The cervical ganglion** sends nerves to the heart, face, neck and eardrum.

> **The celiac ganglion** sends nerves to the adrenal glands, duodenum, kidneys, pancreas and stomach.

> **The splanchnic ganglion** sends nerves to the viscera.

> **The** superior and inferior **mesenteric ganglia** send nerves to the intestines and to the bladder and gonads, respectively.

The parasympathetic ganglia are located in the brain and medulla oblongata: these are the ciliary, optic and sphenopalatine ganglia.

The three levels of peripheral ganglia:

The first ganglion **stage** comprises the paravertebral sympathetic chain.

This chain lies to the side of the vertebral column and extends from the end of the cervical segment to the coccygeal segment.

Located on the sides of the spinal column, it is made up of a series of tiered, interconnected ganglia (paravertebral ganglia) (cervical, thoracic, lumbar and sacral sympathetic ganglia). It is the obligatory transit point for sympathetic fibres to the viscera and glands of the head and neck, thorax, abdomen and pelvis, as well as sympathetic fibres to peripheral somatic regions.

A second lymph node **tier** is made up of pre-visceral nodes or plexuses. They are less numerous than the paravertebral ganglia. They are more like ganglion plexuses than ganglia. They are even and lateral in the neck (carotid, pharyngeal plexuses, etc.) and pelvis, but odd and median in the thorax (cardiac and pulmonary plexuses) and abdomen (solar and lumbo-aortic plexuses).

Pre-visceral ganglia are located close to the viscera. Their role is to gather sympathetic and parasympathetic nerve fibres and distribute them jointly to the nearby viscera (e.g. the celiac ganglia - formerly the solar plexus - distribute their fibres to the viscera of the upper abdomen: liver, stomach, spleen).

A third lymph node **stage** comprises the visceral or terminal lymph nodes located on the surface or in the thickness of the target organ.

c) **The fibres** that connect these levels to each other and to the viscera.

<u>Dermatomes</u>

The spinal column is closely linked to the sympathetic system. The back is an area that is hypersensitive to reflex stimulation, and is linked to **the dermatomes**.

In 1898, Sir H. Head[16] described the distribution of the *dermatome* or cutaneous territory arising from a single posterior, sensitive root. He discovered that pain of visceral origin could be felt on the skin.
Infection, local inflammation, spasm and distension of visceral muscles will lead to cellular suffering.

The dermatome is an area of skin innervated by sensory nerve fibres from a single nerve root. Each spinal nerve emerges from the spinal cord and branches to provide sensations to specific areas of the body. The dermatomes are organised segmentally, following a precise pattern that corresponds to the arrangement of the spinal nerves along the spinal column.

The distribution of dermatomes is systematically mapped in bands covering the whole body. These bands follow a pattern determined by the exit of the spinal nerves from the spinal column. For example, the cervical nerves innervate the skin of the neck and arms, the thoracic nerves innervate the torso, and the lumbar and sacral nerves innervate the legs and feet. Understanding this distribution is crucial for diagnosing certain neurological conditions.

---

[16] Henry Head - Wikipedia (wikipedia.org)

"Everything starts from the central nervous system, made up of the brain and the spinal cord. From the spinal cord, posterior nerve roots (called spinal nerves) descend to each vertebra and then innervate an area of skin: these are the dermatomes," describes Xavier Dufour, physiotherapist. [17]

The dermatomes play an essential role in the transmission of skin sensations to the central nervous system. When a stimulation, such as touch, pain or temperature, occurs on the skin, the sensory receptors in this region send signals through the sensory nerve fibres to the corresponding spinal nerve. The brain interprets these signals to perceive sensations specific to each area of the body.

The visceral functions organise the best possible conditions to serve the musculoskeletal mechanism. They supply and deliver raw materials, including oxygen, as soon as they are consumed. This oxygen, charged with energy, serves as fuel for cell renewal.
Consumed substances must be quickly restored and waste products eliminated to ensure that blood chemistry and homeostasis remain relatively stable. Muscles are the body's largest consumers of energy and the body's economy.

It is the sympathetic (or orthosympathetic) nervous system and the glandular system that are 'responsible', above all for thermoregulation, for adapting visceral, circulatory and metabolic activity to musculoskeletal requirements at all times.

---

[17] Dermatome: definition, usefulness, diagnostic aid (doctissimo.fr)

Reflex techniques help to release muscular and tissue tension, whose imbalances can interfere with nerve impulses and the circulation of blood or fluids.

The plexuses

Everything to do with the sensory and motor systems is linked to the thalamus via the bulb and spinal cord.

Everything to do with major neuro-hormonal control comes through the sympathetic system via secondary relays such as the plexuses and the latero-vertebral chain, coming from the anterior pituitary, which receives fibres from the thalamus via the hypothalamus.

This organisation is monitored and modulated by the parasympathetic system and its ganglia.

The peripheral part of the sympathetic nervous system is characterised by the presence of numerous plexuses.

Plexus: a cluster of intertwined nerves or vessels, ganglionic groupings. They may be nervous, arteriovenous or lymphatic. These plexuses may be the site of an accumulation of internal tension (physical or psychological) giving rise to targeted sensations of unease.

The word plexus is borrowed from the Latin language, and in anatomy designates **a multiple interweaving of several nerve or blood branches** which send ramuscules to each other.

<u>**Nervous plexuses**</u> appear as meshes of varying shapes and sizes, depending on the number of intersecting threads or the layout of the area in which they are placed.

<u>**The main plexuses are :**</u>

- Choroid plexus, in the lateral ventricles of the brain.

- Cervical plexus, on the sides of the neck.

- Brachial plexus: located between the neck and the head of the humerus, it supplies the nerves to the arm.

- The cardiac plexus, behind the aortic arch, is where the cardiac nerves intertwine.

- Pulmonary plexuses, one in front of and one behind the bronchi.

- Solar plexus, on the spine, in the epigastric region.

- The hepatic plexus surrounds the hepatic artery and portal vein.

- Lumbar plexus, in the lower lumbar region.

- Sacral plexus, in front of and below the sacroiliac symphysis.

The celiac, abdominal, lumbar or solar splanchnic plexus is the most important plexus in the abdomen and is the **abdominal vegetative brain.**

<u>**Blood plexuses**</u>: the arterial system, having reached its final limits, can only be seen in the form of plexuses with uneven, tight meshes. There are other venous plexuses which result from the interweaving and anastomosis of branches, as can be seen on the dorsal surfaces of the hand and foot. Their purpose is to facilitate blood circulation in areas exposed to compression.

<u>**Efferent branches**</u> :

They accompany all the branches of the abdominal aorta and supply the sympathetic and vagal contingent to all the abdominal viscera, in the form of <u>secondary plexuses</u>:

 - **The celiac plexus (formerly solar plexus)**: divides into 3 sub-plexuses:

* <u>Gastric</u> or stomachic coronary plexus, destined for the stomach, following the false line of the gastric artery.

* <u>Hepatic</u> plexus, arranged in 2 planes: anterior (satellite of the hepatic artery) and posterior (satellite of the portal vein and bile ducts).

* <u>Splenic</u> plexus, for the duodenum, pancreas, spleen and greater gastric curvature.

 - **The inferior diaphragmatic plexus**: intended for the diaphragmatic dome, without following the arteries.

 - **The adrenal plexus:** comes from the region of the celiac artery and the semilunar ganglion and converges towards the adrenal gland and the upper part of the ureter. It covers the anterior end of the great splanchnic nerve.

- **The renal plexuses:** are arranged peri-arterially and anastomose with the inferior mesenteric plexus.

 - **The superior mesenteric plexus**: destined for the left pancreas, the small intestines and the right colon.

 - **The intermesenteric plexus:** corresponds to the threads which descend in front of and to the sides of the aorta in the interval between the mesenteric arteries. It accompanies the artery and distributes to the left colon and rectum.

- **The spermatic or utero-ovarian plexuses**: satellites of the homonymous arteries, detach from the lower part of the solar plexus. They serve the testicles (men) and adnexa (women).

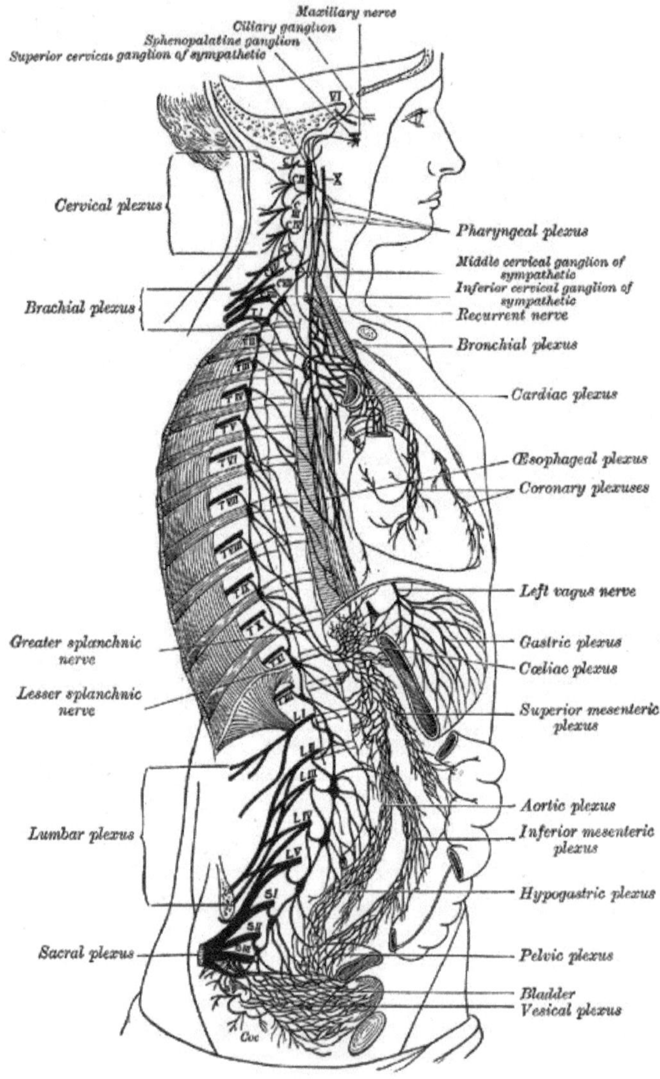

The right sympathetic chain and its connections with the thoracic, abdominal and pelvic plexuses (Schwalbe)

<u>The lymphatic network</u>

The lymphatic system is one of the body's systems for getting rid of impurities. It filters waste and bacteria from the blood.

The circulation of the lymphatic system is dependent on respiratory and muscular movements.

Lymph circulates through the body via a network of vessels that run parallel to the veins.

There are four types:

> ➢ capillaries
> ➢ collecting vessels
> ➢ trunks and
> ➢ canals.

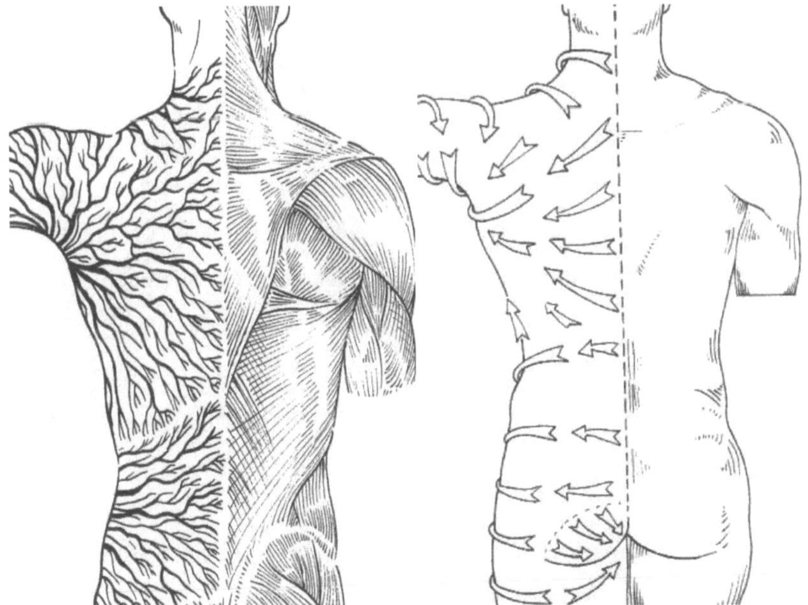

Lymphatic tracts of the trunk - *Posterior surface*
Lympho-Energie® - Drawings by Dominique Jacquemay

The skin

The skin is the body's outer envelope.

The physiological functions of the skin are essential: it is an organ of elimination, an organ of absorption and an organ of perception.

Directly linked to the nervous system, the skin, which contains more than 720,000 nerve endings, conveys sensations and messages, and is our main tool for perceiving the outside world.

The cells of the skin and the nervous system originate from the same layer of the embryo. At the embryological level, the skin, with its **640,000 tactile receptors** connected to the brain and spinal cord, has the same origin (ectodermal) as the neural tube that later gave rise to the Central Nervous System and peripheral nerves.

The skin is the organ of the sense of touch.

The millions of receptors located on the skin, in its tissues and in the sensory zones of our brain enable us to perceive sensations, analyse and interpret signals in the form of pleasant, neutral or unpleasant sensations, recognise cold and heat and react to pain or pressure.

As soon as we place our hands on our body, thousands of receptors come to life to collect sensory information (in this case, pressure through touch will be perceived as a stimulus) and, depending on the "stimuli", different sensory receptors will be excited.

The skin is made up of 3 superimposed layers: the epidermis, the dermis and the hypodermis.

The receptors for touch, which are in fact nerve endings, are found in the skin, and more specifically in its two superficial layers: the epidermis and the dermis. They are particularly abundant on the fingertips, enabling us to explore our environment through touch. Touch is one of our five senses. The sensation of touch is determined by **corpuscles**.

Pacini's corpuscles, the largest (between 1 and 5mm), are located in the deep layers of the dermis, in the aponeuroses of muscles and in the periosteum around joints. They are found in very high concentrations in the fingers and palms of the hands. They enable us to perceive the sense of pressure (baresthesia), when we are tightly wrapped in clothing or shoes, for example.

Meissner corpuscles are much smaller (barely 0.1 mm). They are found mainly on the inside of the hands (palms and underside of fingers) and the soles of the feet. Strictly speaking, these areas are the seat of the tactile sense, enabling us to assess the characteristics of body surfaces.

The so-called Ruffini corpuscles are scattered between the dermis and the epidermis. They inform us of the exact location of a point on the body stimulated by any sensation.

Various sensory receptors in the skin trigger **analgesic and anxiolytic effects**.
The skin also secretes endorphins. It is through these that touch can bring us a feeling of well-being, a soothing, euphoric or regenerative effect. Endorphins are released by the brain (the pituitary gland) during and after the relaxation session. Once released into the bloodstream,

they are dispersed throughout the body, producing their beneficial effects: combating pain, fatigue, anxiety, depression, etc.

Touch also involves another domain, that of OWNERSHIP.

Proprioception enables us to perceive our body and its movements in space, even in the absence of vision. This information, transmitted by the brain, is essential for maintaining balance, managing the strength and direction of our movements and assessing the shape of an object in the hand.

The cerebellum receives all external information: visual, auditory, **tactile,** and information from the body itself: proprioceptive, i.e. kinaesthetic (joints) and muscular (neuromuscular spindles, tendons).
This explains the essential role played by the cerebellum in regulating postural balance.
"Balance is precisely the function that maintains and restores posture at rest and during movement thanks to an appropriate distribution of muscle tone".
The reflexes of the postural muscles are therefore coordinated by the action of the cerebellum, which adjusts the different segments of the body in relation to each other, "defining the position as a whole by processing external and proprioceptive information".

The term somaesthesia can be used as a synonym for sensitivity. It refers to sensitivity to the various stimuli to which the body is subjected - except those originating from the sensory organs - and includes **exteroceptive** sensations (hot, cold, pressure, touch), **nociceptive** sensations (pain) and **proprioceptive** sensations, i.e. those originating from muscles, tendons and joints.

The proprioceptive system is centred in three structures: the spinal cord, the nerves and the brain.
Proprioception enables us to be aware of the position and movements of each part of the body at all times.

This sensitivity is divided into two main parts:
1. **Statesthesia** is the sensation of the position of limbs or body segments in relation to each other and static information.
2. **Kinesthesia** is the sensation of movement that enables us to locate different parts of the body and evaluate their movement (speed and direction).

Each of these two parts, statesthesia and kinesthesia, has its own receptors, **the proprioceptors**, which transmit information to the brain.

1.   **Tendons**: <u>the neurotendinous spindles</u>, also known as Golgi tendon organs, are located at the junction of a tendon and a muscle. Each is formed by a capsule of connective tissue enveloping bundles of collagen fibres.
They protect the tendons and their associated muscles from damage caused by excessive muscular tension. Sensitive to intramuscular tension, they help to regulate muscle stiffness.

2.   **Muscles**: <u>the neuromuscular spindles </u>are located in most skeletal muscles, scattered between and parallel to the myocytes (muscle cells). Each neuromuscular spindle is made up of 3 to 10 specialised myocytes,

enveloped in a connective tissue capsule. The central part of these myocytes contains several sensory nerve endings from the surrounding unipolar neurons. This is the receptor part of the spindles. They measure changes in muscle length and contribute to the stretch reflex.

3.   **Joints**: <u>kinaesthetic receptors </u>(Ruffini, Golgi and Paccini organs). They are located in and around the joint capsules of synovial joints (most joints in the human body). Ruffini's corpuscles and free nerve endings react to pressure; Paccini's corpuscles react to the acceleration and deceleration of the joints during movement.

4.   **Vestibular receptors**: the hair cells of the inner ear also play a role in proprioception. They detect the angular acceleration of rotational movements of the head and signal the linear, vertical or horizontal acceleration of the head and its variations.

All these reflexes (muscular, tissue, vascular, visceral, emotional) modulate our perceptions during reflex massages.
The brain directs our body's internal functions. It weaves links and circuits and also integrates sensory impulses and information to develop perceptions, thoughts and memories.
The brain enables us to be aware of ourselves and gives us the ability to express ourselves and move in our external environment.

By inducing a state of cerebral relaxation, the axis of vigilance is lowered; the sympathetic system is less active and cerebral activity is reduced, leading to a drop in beta waves. The brain no longer needs nerve impulses as much to maintain a state of alertness. The nerve impulses generated by our stimuli are collected in the branches of the autonomic nervous system. This regulates the vital functions of our organs and glands. This is how the reflex regulation coordinated by the autonomic nervous system works.

During the session, there is a **neuronal reorganisation**, allowing an adjustment or rebalancing between the sympathetic and parasympathetic reflexes. There is a kind of survival intelligence in the metabolism that reorganises the rhythms, fluids, movements and intensity of the reflexes of our organs and glands. If, for the survival of the metabolism, the autonomic nervous system considers that an organ or gland needs to reduce or increase its reflex potential, then it will coordinate the sympathetic or parasympathetic reflexes in a very coherent and structured way, according to the needs of the organ or gland in order to maintain the balance and survival of the metabolism.

But this process is operational if the cerebral relaxation has been properly induced beforehand (the lowering of the vigilance axis).
On the other hand, if the vigilance axis is present during the session, the tension in the body (the neuro-musculo-skeletal system) will prevent this neuronal reorganisation of the neuro-vegetative system.
The impact on neurovegetative reflexes will be less, and recovery will be less operational.

PART THREE: BACK REFLEX ZONES

Reflex zones in the back linked to the systems

The back is divided into three main parts: top, middle and bottom.

1. THE TOP OF THE BACK is related to: the nervous system, the endocrine system, the cardiovascular system, the respiratory system and the lymphatic system.

Physically: the sternocleidomastoid muscle, splenius muscle of the head and neck, shoulder lift muscle, deltoid muscle, trapezius muscle, trapezius tendon.

Linked to the vigilance axis and neuro-hormonal circuits.

2. THE BACK ENVIRONMENT is related to: the cardiovascular system, the respiratory system, the digestive system and the lymphatic system.

Physically: the dorsalis major muscle, rhomboid muscle, posterosuperior and posteroinferior serratus muscles, thoracolumbar fascia.

Linked to the solar plexus (emotional).

3. THE BOTTOM OF THE BACK is related to: the urogenital system.

Physically: the oblique muscle, quadratus lumborum, gluteal fascia, gluteus medius muscle, gluteus maximus muscle, multifidus muscles, lumbosacral fascia.

Linked to the elimination system.

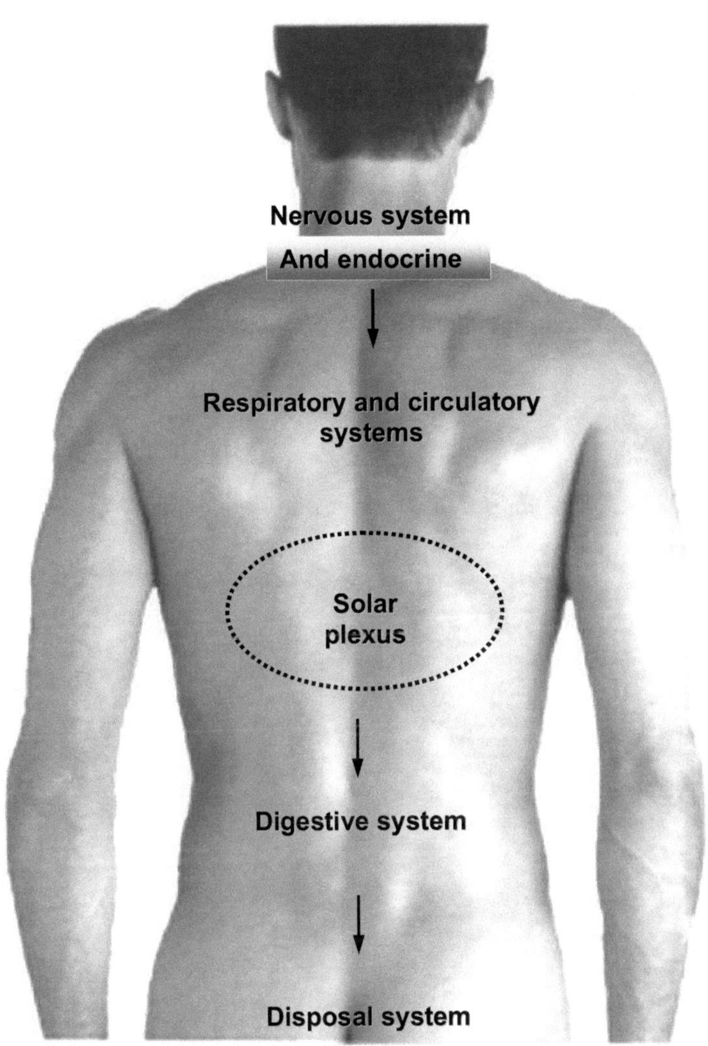

Nervous system
And endocrine
Respiratory and circulatory
systems
Solar
plexus
Digestive system
Disposal system

<u>**Reflex zones in the back linked to organs and glands**</u>

UPPER BACK :

Brain, thyroid and parathyroid glands, larynx, pharynx, cervical vertebrae, shoulders, elbows, arms, trapezius.

THE MIDDLE OF THE BACK :

Lungs, heart, thymus, oesophagus, stomach, large and small intestines, colon, liver, gall bladder, pancreas, spleen, appendix, dorsal and lumbar vertebrae.

LOWER BACK :

Adrenal glands, kidneys, ureter, bladder and genitourinary organs, colon and rectum.

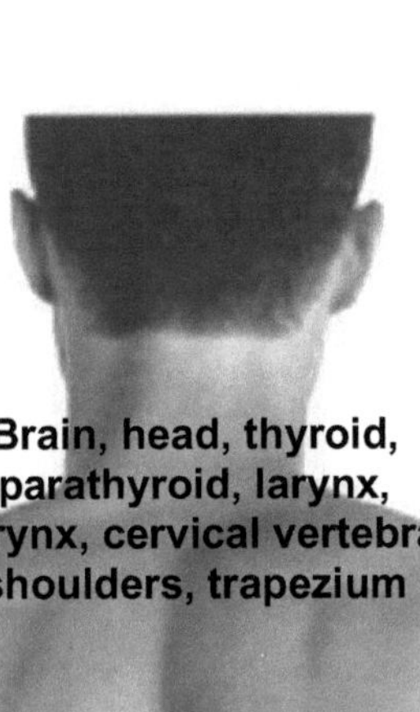

Brain, head, thyroid, parathyroid, larynx, pharynx, cervical vertebrae, shoulders, trapezium
Lungs, heart, thymus, sternum, oesophagus, stomach, diaphragm, dorsal vertebrae
Kidneys, adrenal glands, small intestine, large intestine, colon, gall bladder, liver, pancreas, spleen, lumbar vertebrae
Colon, rectum, reproductive organs, bladder, Sacrum and coccyx

<u>**Case studies**</u>

Since 2015, I have been taking part in scientific conferences (AMEC, GETCOP, ICEPS, NPIS) where I present our research and observational studies.

At the "*3rd GETCOP Thematic Days - Chronic lumbago and manual therapies*" conference, held on 18 and 19 June 2021 in Nancy[18] , I presented three posters, which are shown below.

1[er] poster entitled :

Chronic lumbago and connective, periosteal and viscerocutaneous reflex techniques *(osteopathic contribution to reflexology)*®

Introduction

Several hundred subjects of both sexes, with no clinical diagnosis or contraindication to reflex massage of the back, have been treated for low back pain and monitored in reflexology practices since 2002. Most of them suffered from anxiety, back pain and chronic low back pain due to stress.

Psychological factors, including emotional stress, can predispose, precipitate or aggravate low back pain. They encourage the onset of chronicity and form part of the psychosocial indicators known as "yellow flags".

The method applied

---

[18] Chronic lumbago and manual therapies - 3rd Thematic Days of GETCOP GETCOP - Groupe d'Évaluation des Thérapies Complémentaires Personnalisées (Group for the Evaluation of Personalised Complementary Therapies) % %

Theoretical basis

Conjunctival, periosteal and viscerocutaneous reflex techniques aim to :

> ➤ reduce sympathetic hyperactivity in functional disorders, joint and muscle pain, etc.
> ➤ drain connective tissue
> ➤ restore and maintain metabolic homeostasis.

Method

Connective, periosteal and viscerocutaneous reflex techniques (reflex massage of connective tissue in the back).

Stress causes hyperfunction of the nervous system and hypertonicity of the musculoskeletal system, particularly in the back. The back is an area that is hypersensitive to reflex stimulation, and is linked to the dermatomes. Stimulation of the muscle and ligament receptors in the different muscle layers of the back, as well as the different skin corpuscles, leads to muscle relaxation and the secretion of well-being hormones (endorphin, dopamine, etc.).

Reflex stimulation of the connective tissue decongests the treated area locally and acts at a distance (derivative effect).

Research objective

To evaluate the results of a reflexology practice in a more objective way than the satisfaction expressed by people with low back pain.

Materials and method

We have collated, on a case-by-case basis, some twenty years of observations: an observational approach within the framework and with the limited resources of daily practice in a reflexology clinic.

Protocol and procedure

Observation survey carried out by myself and people trained in my method (around 200 practitioners).

An average of three to five sessions of reflex massage of the connective tissue of the back were given once a month.

Criteria for judging results

Pain and stress assessment scales, before and after back reflex treatment. Photographs were also taken to monitor the evolution and tissue changes of the back, and the various local skin reactions: rubefactions, bulges, etc.

Results / Discussion

From one session to the next, we observed and noted greater tissue relaxation, less pain, less fatigue, a significant drop in nervous tension, as well as muscular and postural changes producing a greater sense of well-being. This also had a positive impact on the mind, with better management of pain and emotions.

Conclusion

This collection of observations suggests that reflex massage of the back is an interesting indication for the treatment of low back pain caused by emotional stress.

<u>2 poster entitled</u> :

The contribution of Reflex Techniques for the back in supporting a person weakened by bereavement

Introduction :

Grief is a reaction and a feeling of sadness experienced following the death of a loved one. Often associated with suffering and causing emotional stress, this state causes hyperfunction of the sympathetic nervous system, hypertonia of the musculoskeletal system and, in particular, a great deal of tension in the back. Reflex techniques for the back bring about changes in the tissues, muscles and posture, as well as calming the emotions.

Method :

Connective, periosteal and viscerocutaneous reflex techniques (reflex massage of connective tissue in the back).

Case study :

Mrs V.G., aged 38, received six sessions from October 2009 to April 2010, following an emotional shock (death of her mother). She was complaining of back pain and stiffness, similar to a 'bar' in the lumbar region, with an unexpressed, suppressed emotional overload. Her back is congested, slightly swollen, with a redder colouration, and the skin is sensitive to touch. She has no clinical diagnosis and no contraindications to back reflex techniques.

Number of back reflex massage sessions: 6.
One session per month except February.

1.   10/10/2009
2.   07/11/2009
3.   05/12/2009
4.   09/01/2010
5.   13/03/2010
6.   10/04/2010

Results :

Photos were taken before and after the dorsal reflex treatment in order to compare the evolution and tissue changes of the back, and the different local skin reactions: rubefactions, bulges, etc.

Over the course of the sessions, her back changed its appearance and texture, both physically (significant changes in the connective tissue, *"a back that deflated, that breathed"*, as V.G. put it) and psychologically (gradual release of her emotional state, a feeling that she had emptied herself, freed of a *"heavy weight"*...).

Subject: V.G. (38 years old, sex F)

Protocol: BACK REFLEX MASSAGE

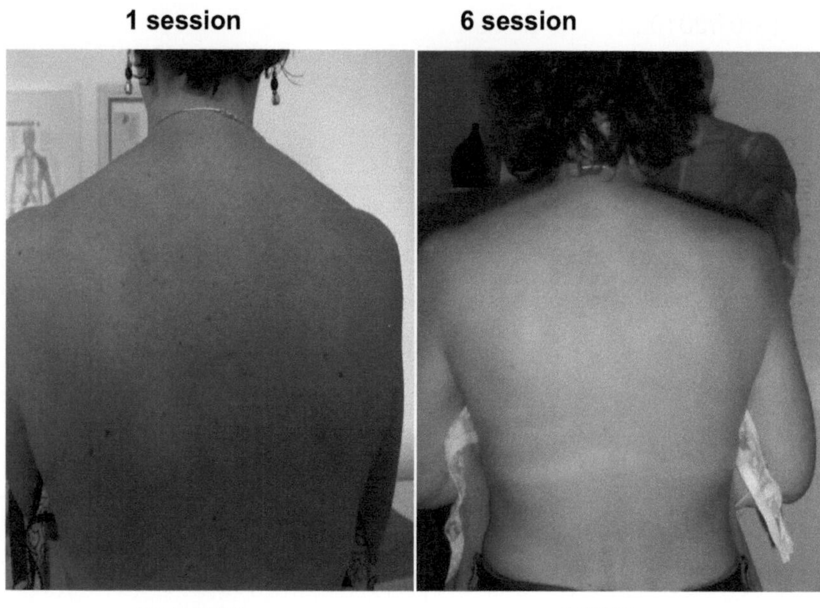

Conclusion:

Regular reflex massages brought about changes in the subject's tissues, muscles and posture. There was also a positive impact on the mind and better management of pain and emotions.

<u>3 poster entitled</u> :

The contribution of back reflex techniques to pain management in people with disc disease

Introduction :

A.B. suffers from L5-S1 degenerative disc disease from time to time, as revealed by MRI. Excessive strain, such as carrying heavy loads, can trigger pain and provoke an "acute attack".

Method :

Connective, periosteal and viscerocutaneous reflex techniques (reflex massage of connective tissue in the back).

Case study :

Mrs A.B., aged 23, received five sessions (one session a day), over the course of a week, following the "reawakening" of back pain caused by carrying heavy loads (temporary manual work in a large shopping centre).

Visual Analogue Scale: Use of the VAS scale before and after the dorsal reflex treatment. This scale measures pain intensity on a scale from 0 to 10.

Results :

Subject: A.B. (23 years old, sex F)

Protocol: BACK REFLEX MASSAGE

	date	Level of pain BEFORE	Level of pain AFTER
1st session	02/04/2021	9	8
2nd session	03/04/2021	8	5
3rd session	04/04/2021	5	4
4th session	05/04/2021	4	3
5th session	13/04/2021	2	1

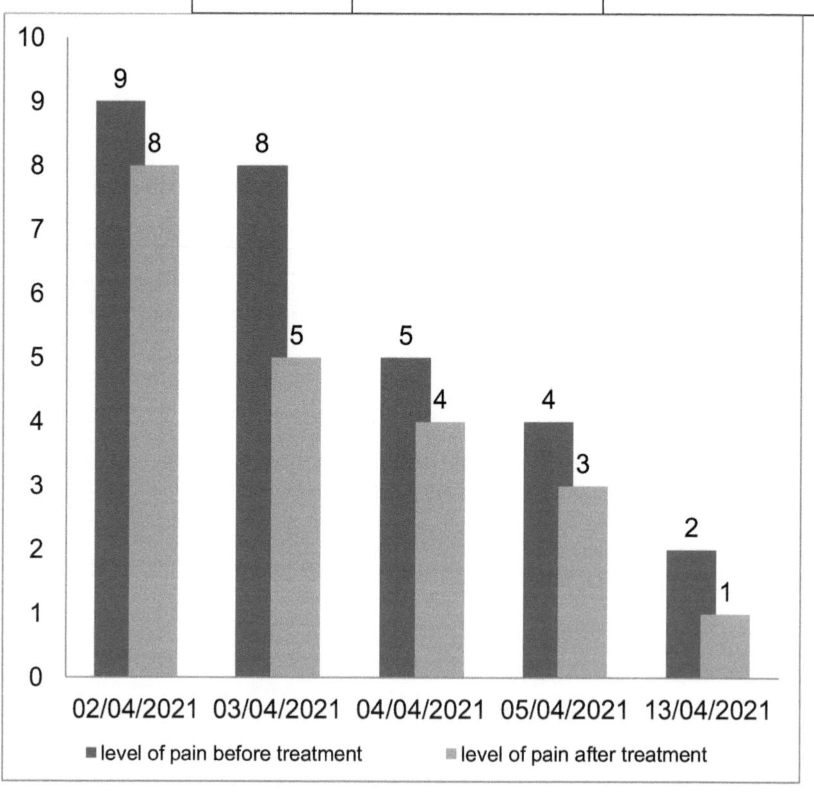

Exceptionally, I followed the A.B. subject over 4 affiliate days. We spaced out the 5th (last) session, but on the whole, the five sessions were very close together.

As a general rule, back reflex massage sessions can be offered every 3 weeks. This is a rhythm that allows you to follow the evolution and progressive transformations of the connective tissue of the back.
The results are often immediate from the first session onwards (less tissue congestion, less tightness, less tension, less pain, etc.).
People feel relieved, breathe more easily and have a fuller diaphragm. They say they feel as if a weight has been lifted, a burden has been lifted, and they feel calmer and more serene.

***

These posters have been published in the journal HEGEL and posted on the CAIRN.INFO platform.
➢   The contribution of back reflex techniques to pain management in people with disc disease
https://www.cairn.info/revue-hegel-2021-3-page-288.htm
➢   Chronic lumbago and connective, periosteal and viscerocutaneous reflex techniques
https://www.cairn.info/revue-hegel-2021-3-page-293.htm

Subject L.M. (aged 50, sex F)

Protocol: BACK REFLEX MASSAGE

<u>Only 1 session was carried out</u> on 24/02/2022

The back BEFORE the session

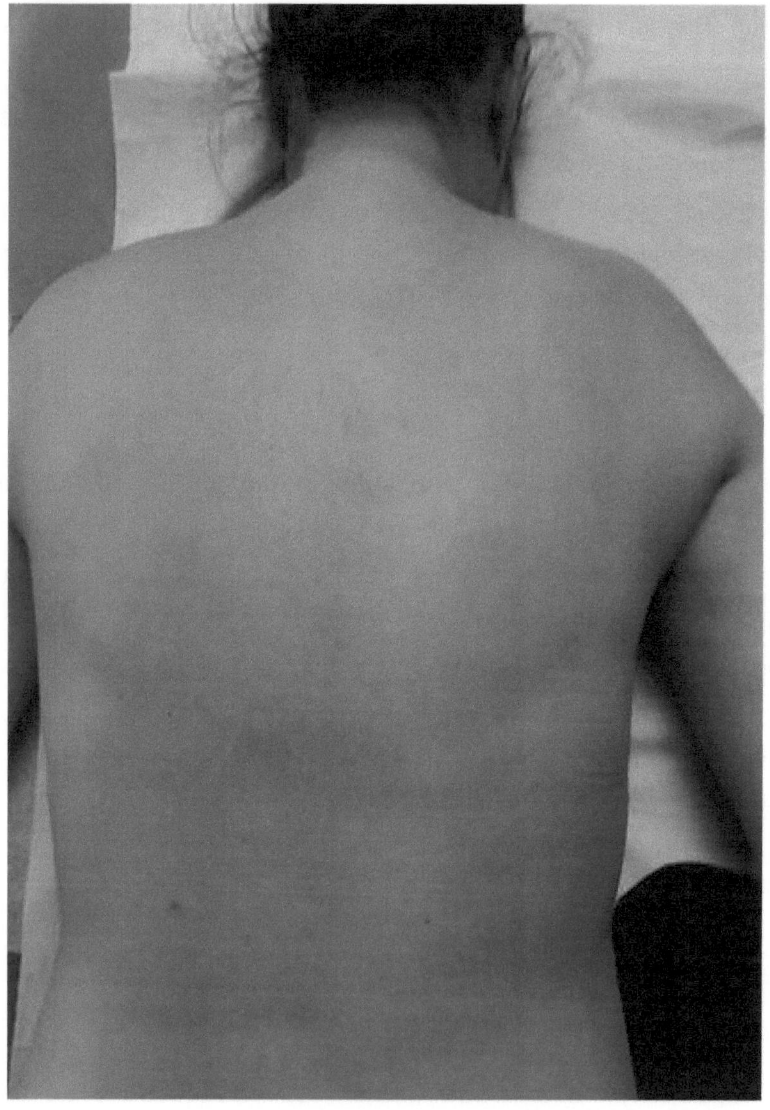

After 30 minutes of reflex back massage, there was a significant change in the upper back, a "deflation" of the tissue between the shoulder blades. And a "slimming" of the waist.

The back AFTER the session

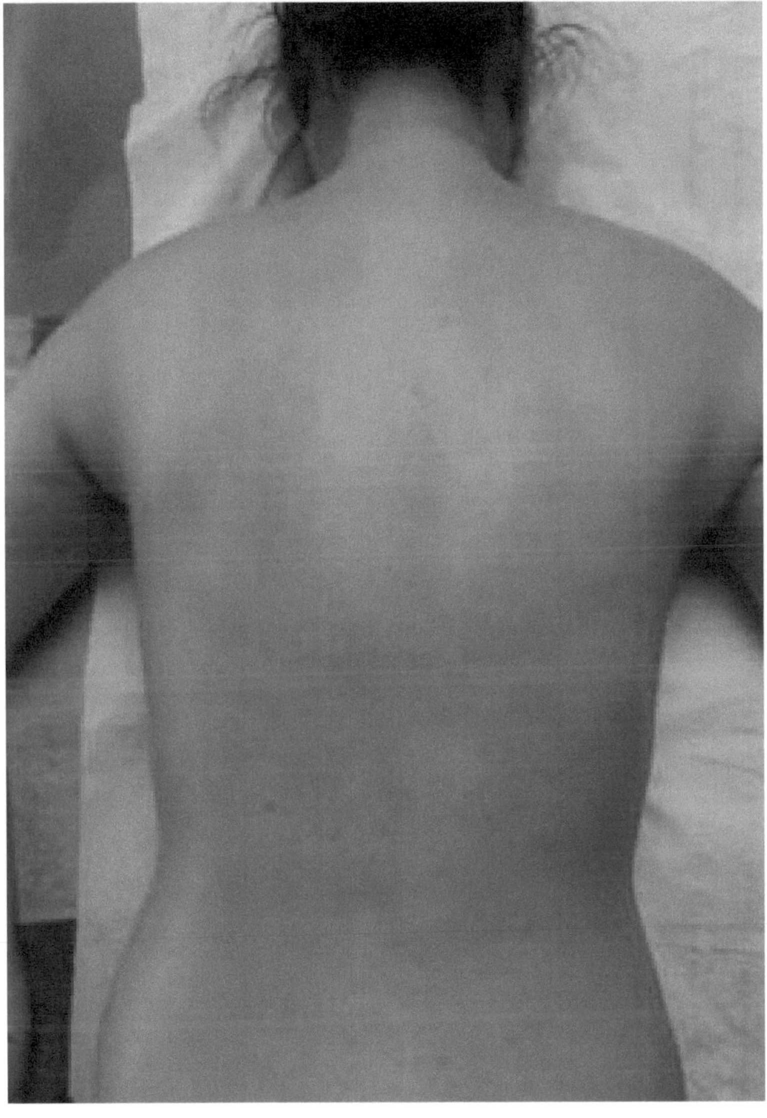

PHOTO CONTINUATION

Subject L.M. (aged 50, sex F)

Protocol: BACK REFLEX MASSAGE

<u>Only 1 session </u>was carried out on 24/02/2022

The back BEFORE the session

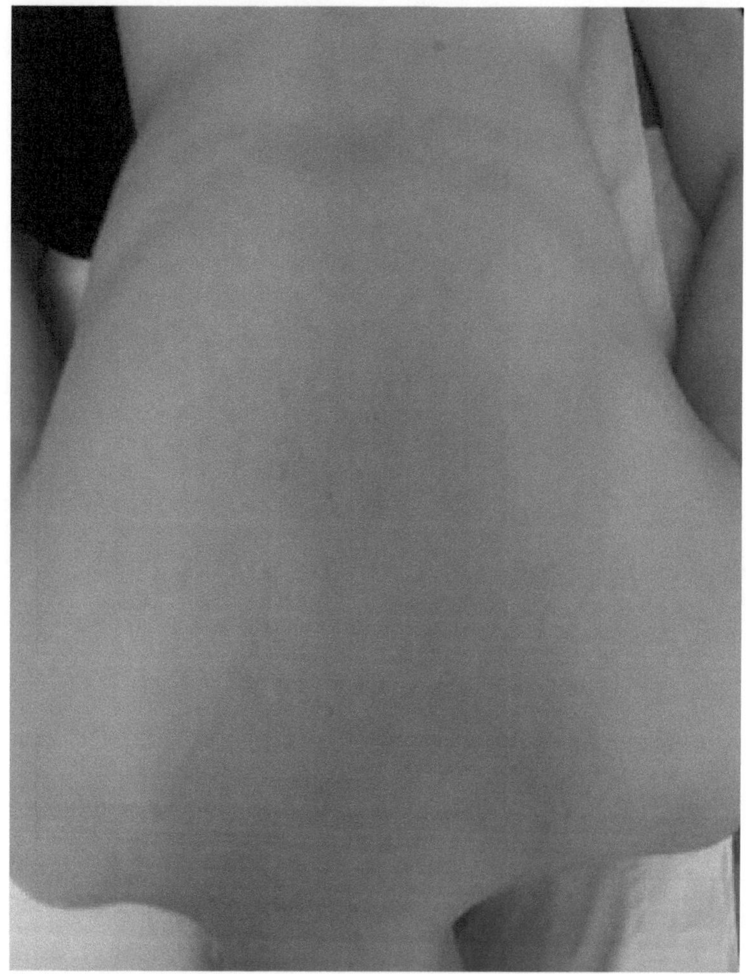

After 30 minutes of reflex massage of the back, the back felt slimmer, as if it had been lengthened. In the photo, you can see a better fit and symmetry at the waist, towards the lower back.

The back AFTER the session

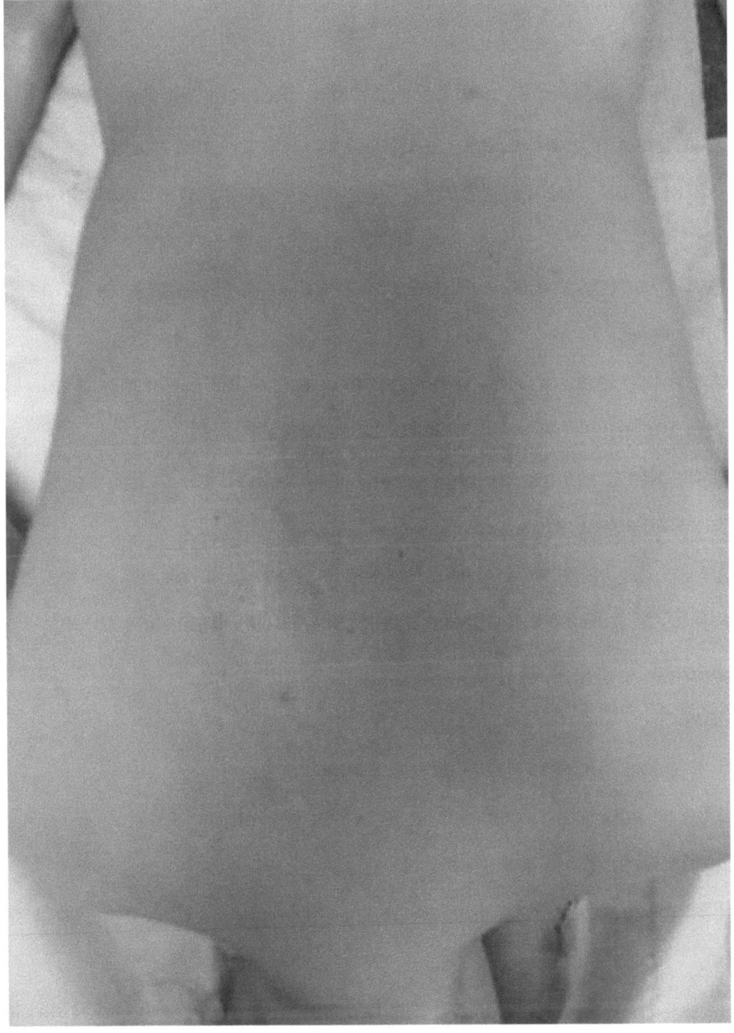

Protocol - reflex back massage

Before you start

- To practise back reflex relaxation properly, it is advisable to have a minimum knowledge of the anatomy and physiology of the human body, and experience of reflex touch.

- Respect your limits and do not make medical diagnoses.

- Carry out a brief check-up by asking the person about their state of health and their history (illness, operation, scarring, medication taken, treatment in progress, etc.).

- Avoid practising on subjects with serious illnesses (or undergoing chemotherapy).

- As a precaution, and if necessary, refer the person to their GP or any other therapist (physiotherapist or osteopath).

- If it's the first time, explain that reflex relaxation of the back relaxes the body and eliminates tissue toxins.

- Warn the person that it is necessary to drink plenty of water after the session to further encourage the process of eliminating toxins.

- Inform them that they may feel a little tired or sore after the session.

- It is advisable to rest after the session.

- Make sure the subject has removed their belt and jewellery (necklaces, bracelets, watch, etc.).

- Make sure they are able to lie on their stomach to benefit from the session.

- Make sure the room is at the right temperature. A cold room is not conducive to relaxation.

-       The session takes place in a calm environment, and can be accompanied by soft, pleasant music.

-       Keep a bottle of oil for application, wipes and a blanket to cover the person close at hand.

-       You should be calm and relaxed. Without rings or bracelets, with clean, well-cut nails, and dressed comfortably for the session.

-       The session can last from 20 to 30 minutes maximum, the movements are firm and gentle, wide and deep.

-       After the back reflex relaxation session, you can follow up with other reflex relaxation techniques (plantar, palmar, facial or auricular).

<u>NOTE</u> :

The study and knowledge of the main systems of the human body are essential to the practice and to the acquisition of a better physical and physiological understanding of metabolism.

For a better application of the protocol and method, and to master the reflex touch, it is recommended to follow the teaching offered at the Elisabeth Breton Training Centre.

Reflex back massage protocol (Elisabeth Breton method)

First manoeuvre
Contact is made with the person by smoothing the entire back, first dry and then with the application of massage oil.

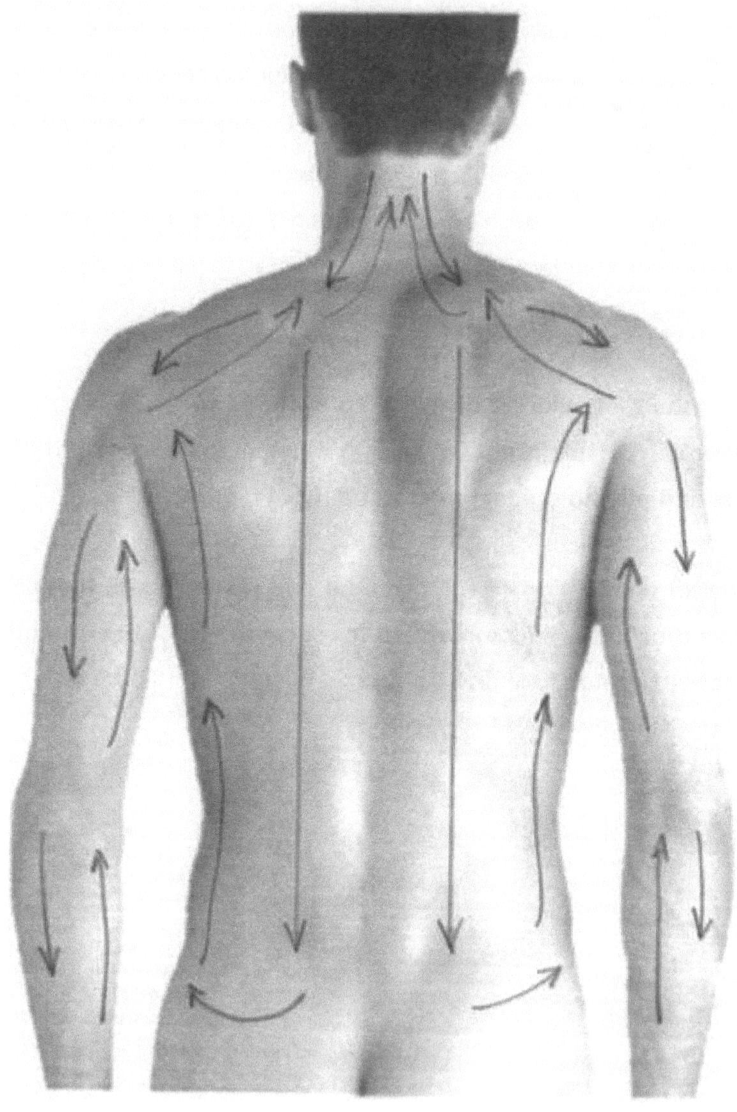

Second manoeuvre

Smooth one side of the back, then the other, passing through the arm to the thumb. Manoeuvre from the lower back (quadratus lumborum) upwards (scapula lift), one side then the other.

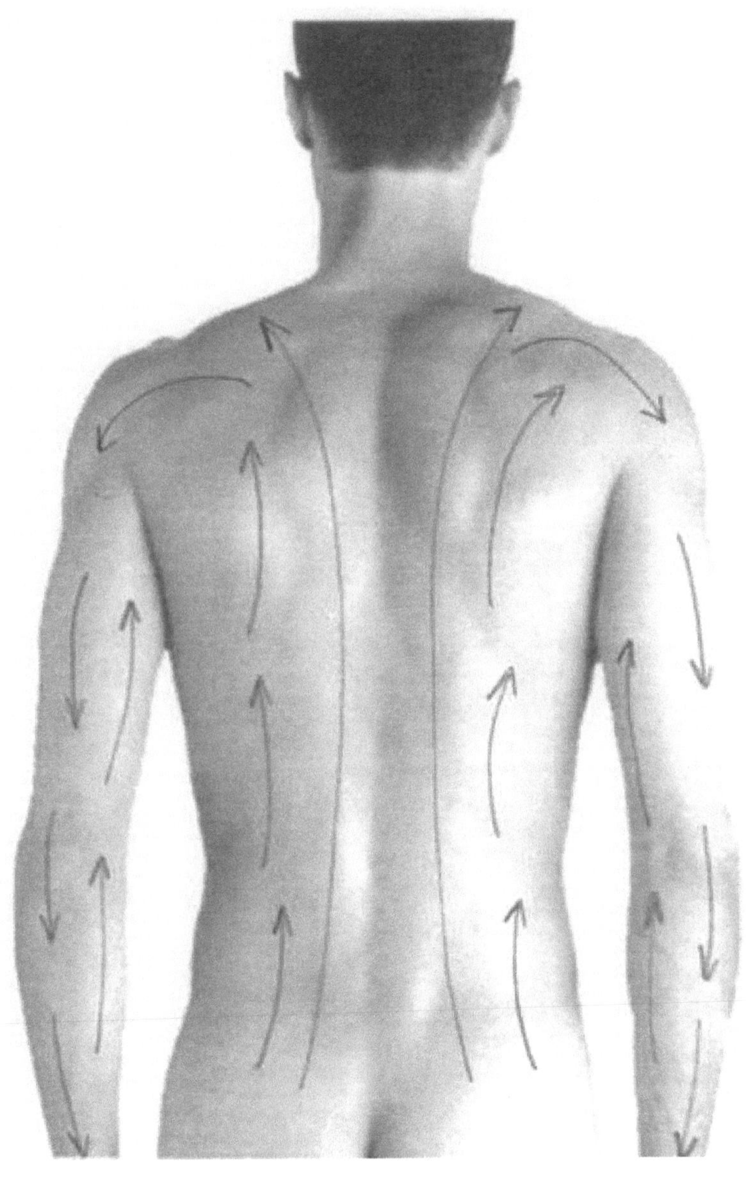

Third manoeuvre

Big movement of the complete smoothing of the back. Like the first movement. Manoeuvres from the top (starting from the nape of the neck) downwards (sacrum).

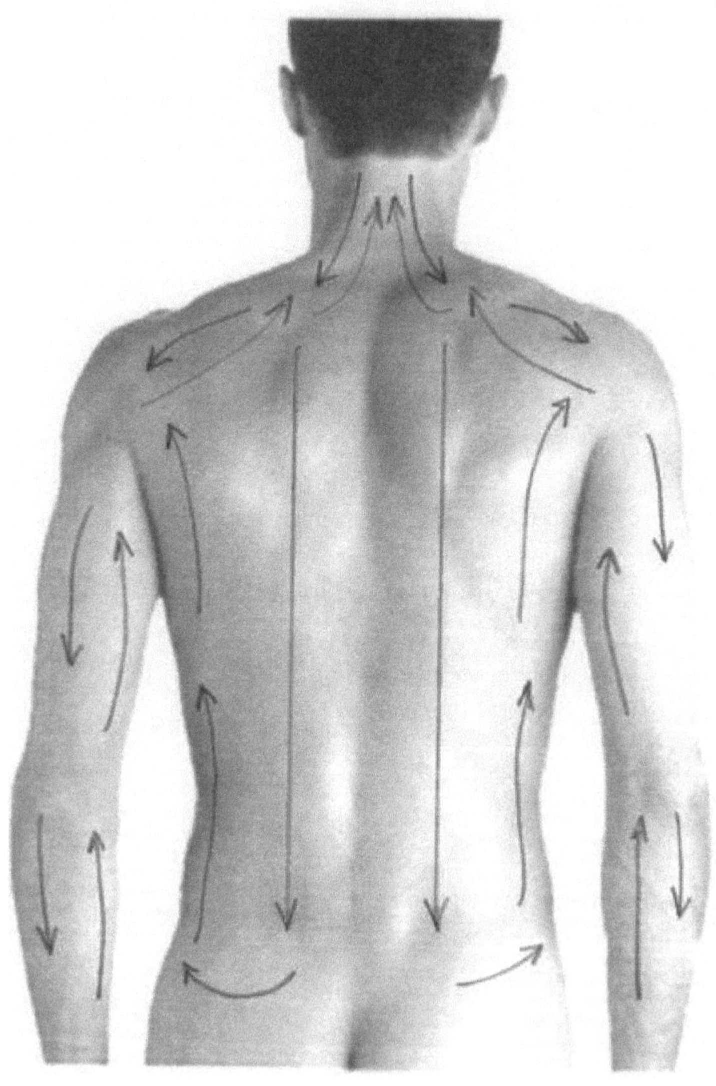

Fourth manoeuvre
Carry out a "gentle detachment" of the connective tissue, moving down simultaneously and on both sides of the spinal column.
Relaxation of the splenius muscles of the head and neck, trapezius, long dorsalis, multifidus muscles, the transversalis spinae.
Relaxation of the thoracolumbar fascia and lumbosacral fascia.
Working upwards from the bottom, grasp the outer edges of the body.

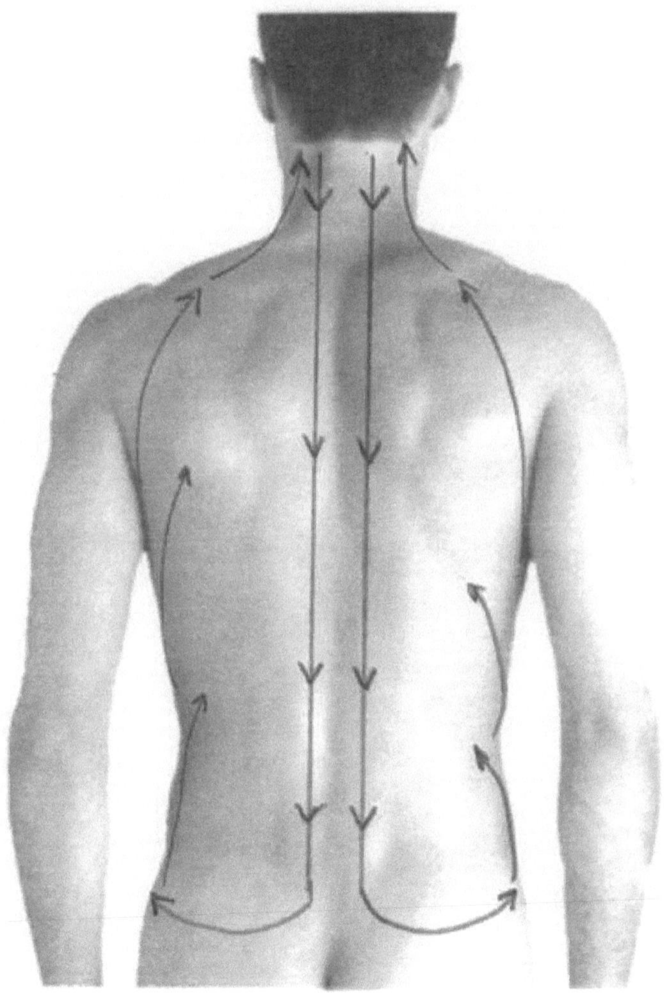

Fifth manoeuvre

Repetition of the first movement (like the third).
Great back smoothing.

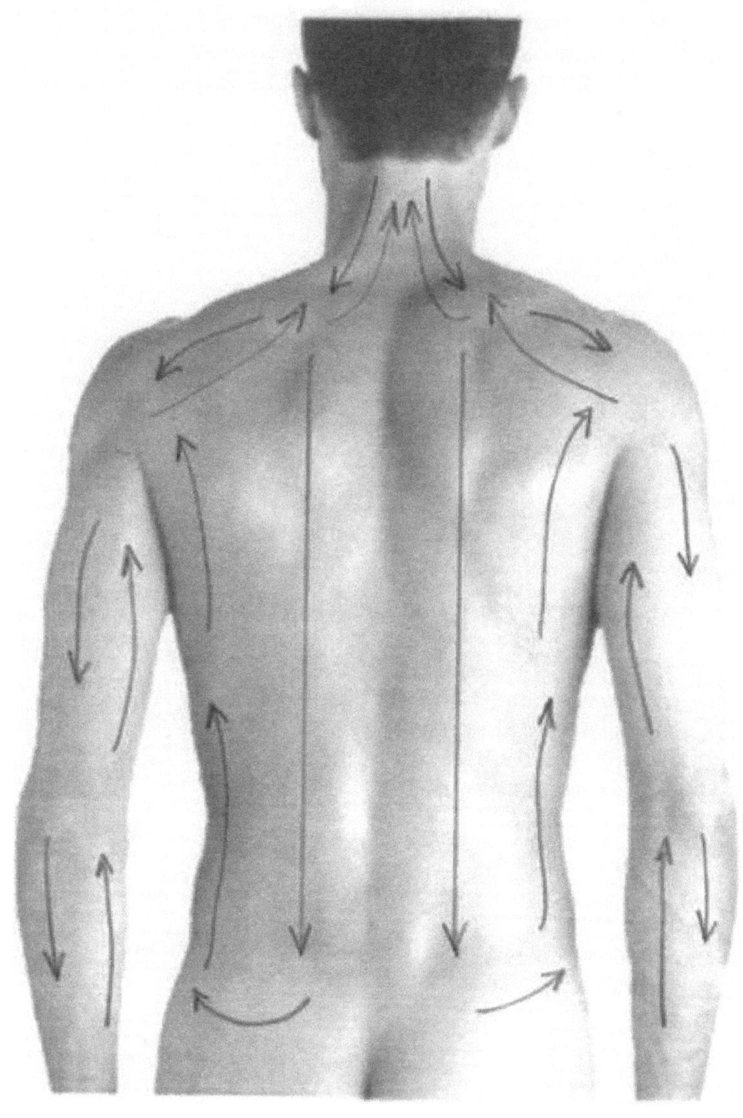

Sixth manoeuvre
Work on the upper back (drainage of the shoulder girdle: shoulders, shoulder blades, trapezius). Then the ribs (the intercostal spaces), followed by the squared lumbar muscles, oblique muscles, flank, and move upwards with small rotating movements, from the pelvis towards the nape of the neck, the edge of one side, then apply the same manoeuvres to the other side.

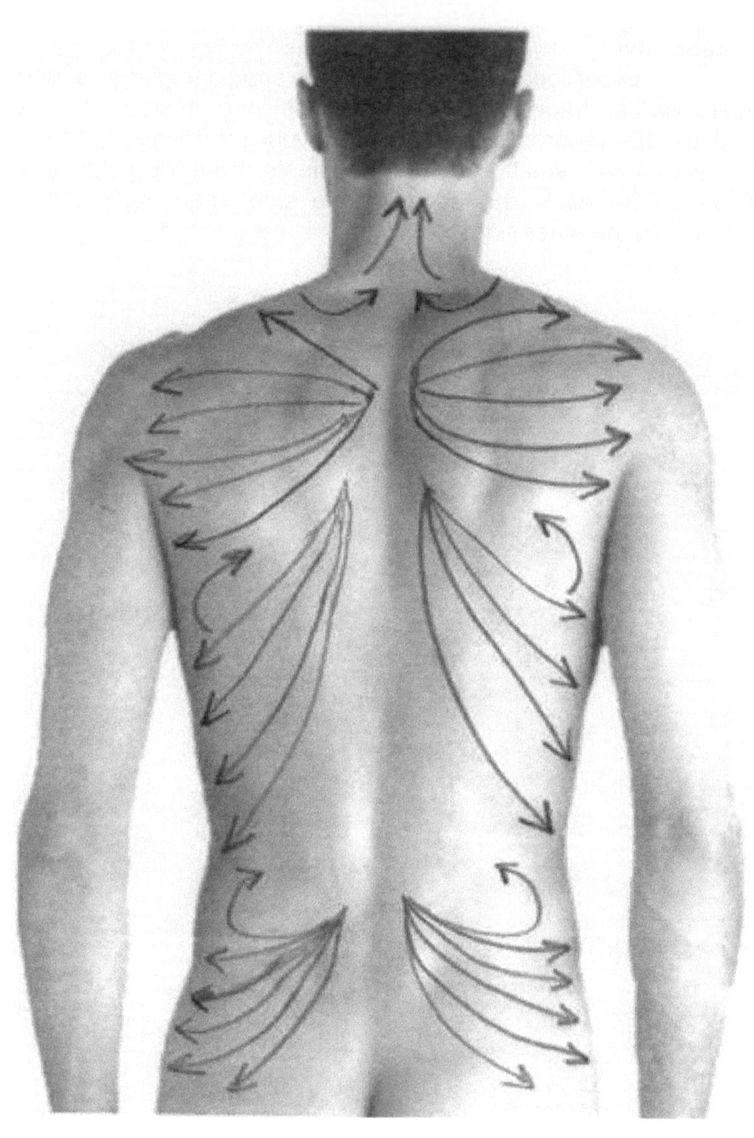

Repetition of the first movement (like the 3rd and 5th).
Great back smoothing.

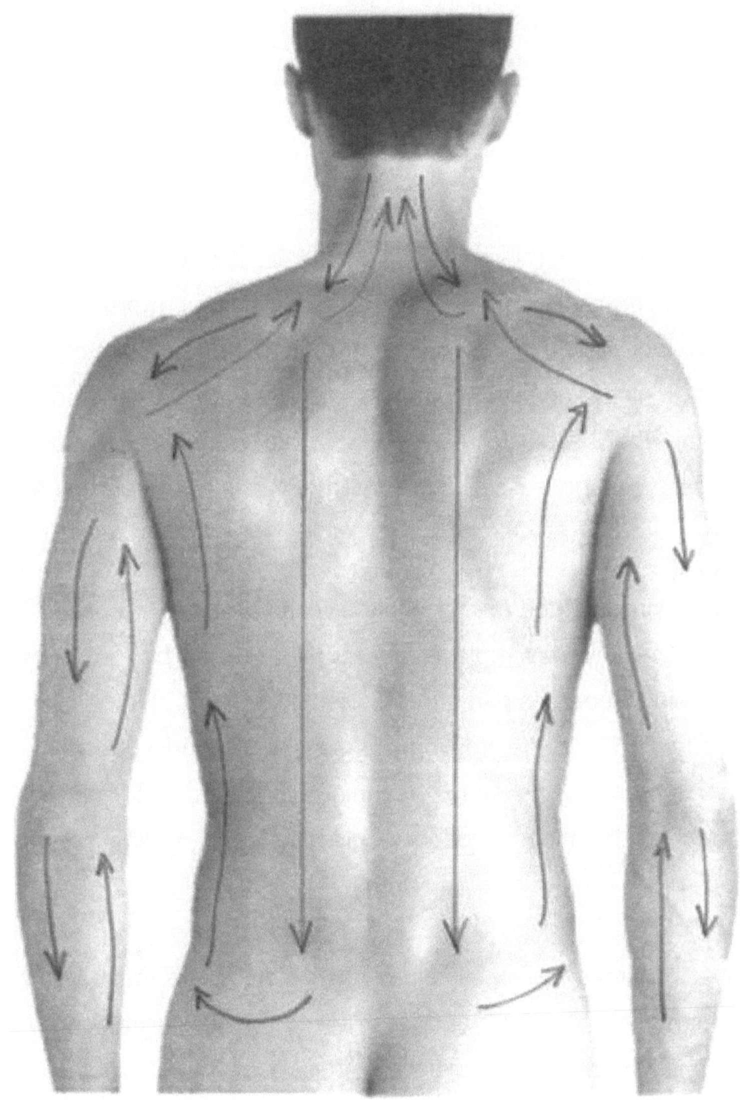

<u>**Last movement**</u>

Cover the person and press lightly on their back.
Place one hand on the nape of the neck/tendon of the trapezius (cervical plexus) and the other on the sacrum (sacral plexus).
Stay like this for a few minutes.
Then apply gentle pressure around the body.

***

<u>**Note to readers**</u>

In no way does the information provided in this book constitute a recommendation for treatment (preventive or curative), a prescription or a diagnosis, nor should it be considered as such. In the event of serious discomfort or illness, you should first consult a doctor or healthcare professional who is able to assess your state of health appropriately. Reflexology massage sessions are intended solely for relaxation and well-being.

The information provided in this book is for information purposes only. They do not in any way replace the courses offered by the Elisabeth Breton Training Centre as part of professional training.
It is important to follow a training course focusing on supporting and caring for people using reflex techniques, in order to obtain the professional qualifications needed to practise as a relaxologist and/or reflexologist.

The relaxation and/or reflex stimulation protocols in this manual are the fruit of many years' work, and are based on the experience and exchanges of practice of practitioners trained at the Elisabeth Breton Training Centre.

Indications and contraindications

Indications:

- ➢ Relaxes tissues, muscles and nerves by releasing tension.
- ➢ Improves blood microcirculation.
- ➢ Tissue drainage and elimination of toxins.
- ➢ Increased levels of endorphins and improved nerve impulses.
- ➢ Release from emotional stress.

Contraindications:

- ➢ Serious infection and illness accompanied by high fever
- ➢ Inflammatory process affecting the venous and lymphatic system
- ➢ Pregnancy at risk, the first 3 months of pregnancy
- ➢ Cancer (risk of dispersed outbreaks)
- ➢ Wearers of pacemakers or stants

Take care with fragile individuals: children, pregnant women and the elderly.

CONCLUSION

These days, health problems are often linked to **stress**. A well-rested person suffers less from exhaustion and fatigue, and is less sensitive to stress.

The more sensitive our hands become, the more we realise that healthy muscles feel elastic, supple, soft, warm and alive, whereas a tense muscle feels harder, drier, colder and denser to the touch.

Reflex massage of the back gradually brings about general relaxation of all the muscular layers, from the superficial to the deep levels, and releases the emotional stress accumulated in the connective tissue of the back, reducing physical and emotional tension.

** These services are not medical in nature and are in no way intended to replace medical treatment or prescriptions for medication.*
** Sessions are not a substitute for treatment by physiotherapists or osteopaths.*
** Sessions are aimed solely at stress prevention and management, relaxation and well-being.*

BIOGRAPHY OF THE AUTHOR

Elisabeth Breton, a criminologist by training, has been working in the field of prevention, stress management and personal well-being since 2001. She specialises in relaxation and stimulation reflex techniques derived from osteopathy, and offers relaxologist and reflexologist training courses.

In 2015, her training centre became the first certifier for the RNCP (Répertoire national des certifications professionnelles) reflexology qualification[19] .

Elisabeth Breton is co-founder of the Collégiale des fédérations et des syndicats de réflexologie . [20]

In 2023, she initiated the AFNOR standard project on reflexology service quality[21] .

Elisabeth Breton is president of the "La Fontaine du Bien-être" association, and a member of the :

- ➢ the Pain and the Painful Patient Association (LDPD)
- ➢ the Association of RNCP Reflexologists (ARRNCP),
- ➢ of the Citizen Network of the MCA Agency (RC-AMCA)
- ➢ the Evaluation Group for Personalised Complementary Therapies (GETCOP)
- ➢ of the Chamber of Sustainable Health Practitioners
- ➢ of the Association Française de Criminologie and the Association Internationale des Criminologues de Langue Française.

---

[19] Arrêté du 17 juillet 2015 portant enregistrement au répertoire national des certifications professionnelles - Légifrance (legifrance.gouv.fr)

[20] Collegiale des Fédérations & Syndicats de la Réflexologie - Together to go further (collegiale-federations-syndicats-reflexologie.com)

[21] Structure AFNOR/S99R | Norm'Info

Elisabeth Breton specialises in :

> Stress and Anxiety Management, at SYMBIOFI (Interactive
Emotional Self-Therapy, Innovative Solutions for Stress), a partner
of the Lille University Hospital Centre.
> Medical Stress Management, at AEMI (European Academy of
Integrative Medicine).

Since 2015, she has taken part in the scientific conferences of:
> Anti-aging Medicine European Congress (AMEC)
> Group for the Evaluation of Personalised Complementary
Therapies (GETCOP)
> Non-Medication Interventions (ICEPS, NPIS)

Elisabeth Breton is co-author and author of several books on reflexology
and stress.

BIBLIOGRAPHY

Amoyel J. " La médecine manuelle", Editions Dangles, 1989.

Breton E., Réflexologie pour la forme et le bien-être, Editions Vie, 2014.

Breton E., Facial and cranial reflexology, Editions Vie, 2015.

Breton E., Réflexologie, un vrai remède au stress, Editions Vie, 2015.

Breton E., Valéro J., Le stress, ça vous parle? Comprendre son histoire et ses mécanismes, Editions Vie, 2021.

Breton E, Valéro J., Réflexologie et troubles fonctionnels, DUNOD, 2022.

Eschalier I., La fasciathérapie - Une nouvelle méthode pour le bien-être ", Edition Point d'Appui.

Richard R., Techniques réflexes conjonctives, périostées et dermalgies viscéro cutanées, Richard's Osteopathic Research Institute (RORI) 2001.

<u>SITOGRAPHY</u>

Elisabeth Beton Training Centre
www.reflexobreton.fr

Association La Fontaine du Bien-être
http://www.fontainedubienetre.fr/

Pain and the Painful Patient Association
http://www.la-douleur-et-le-patient-douloureux.fr/Accueil/accueil.php

Association of RNCP Reflexologists (ARRNCP)
https://www.reflexologues-rncp.com/

Collégiale des Fédérations et des Syndicats de la Réflexologie
https://collegiale-federations-syndicats-reflexologie.com/

Réseau Citoyen-Agence Médecine Complémentaire et Adaptées
https://www.agencemca.fr/

National Office for Information on Education and Careers (ONISEP)
https://www.onisep.fr

NON-PHARMACOLOGICAL INTERVENTION SOCIETY (NPIS)
https://npisociety.org/

Evaluation Group for Personalised Complementary Therapies
http://congres-therapiescomplementaires.org/getcop_home.php
The Chamber of Sustainable Health Professions

http://www.chambre-professions-sante-durable.fr/

Stress Prevention and Management
https://www.preventiongestionstress.com/

Psycho&Bien-être, Portal for Psycho, Health and Wellbeing
http://www.psycho-bien-etre.be/bien-etre/reflexologie

Treating stress: new tools, new approaches www.symbiofi.com

HANTONE® - Support for vulnerable people https://www.hantone.fr/

ReflexoXP Software - Home - ReflexoXP

Le Point Réflexe - Magazine
https://www.reflexesante.ch/magazine

ICAMAR - Medical journal on auriculotherapy and auricular acupressure
http://www.icamar.org

HEGEL - Scientific and medical journal
https://www.cairn.info/revue-hegel.htm

CAIRN.INFO - Digital library in the humanities and social sciences
Welcome | Cairn.info
NUMETIK AVOCATS
https://www.numetik-avocats.fr/

UPGCS

Union for the Prevention and Management of Health Crises
UPGCS HEALTH ALERT - UPGCS Health Crisis Alerts

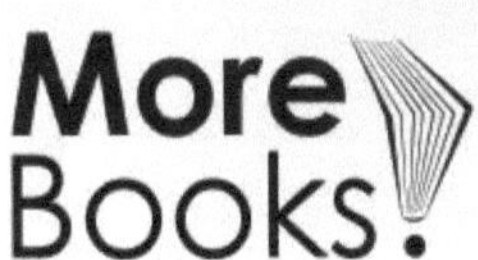

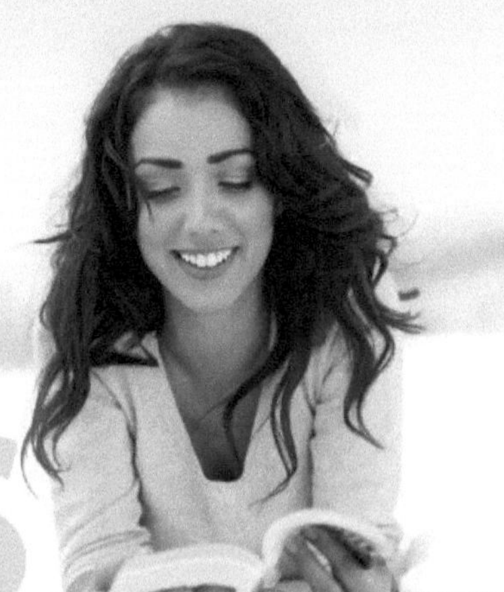

I want morebooks!

Buy your books fast and straightforward online - at one of world's fastest growing online book stores! Environmentally sound due to Print-on-Demand technologies.

Buy your books online at
www.morebooks.shop

Kaufen Sie Ihre Bücher schnell und unkompliziert online – auf einer der am schnellsten wachsenden Buchhandelsplattformen weltweit! Dank Print-On-Demand umwelt- und ressourcenschonend produzi ert.

Bücher schneller online kaufen
www.morebooks.shop

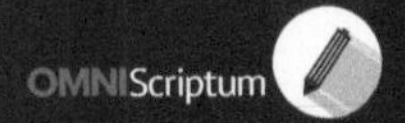

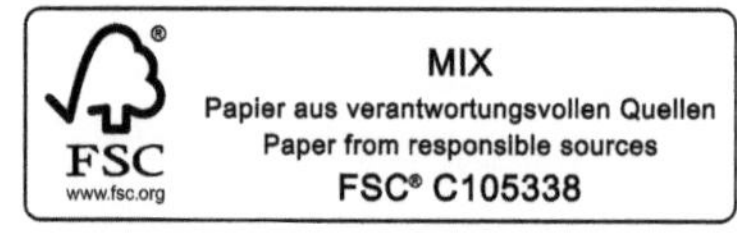

Printed by Books on Demand GmbH, Norderstedt / Germany